Also Available From the American Academy of Pediatrics

Common Conditions

ADHD: What Every Parent Needs to Know

Allergies and Asthma: What Every Parent Needs to Know

My Child Is Sick! Expert Advice for Managing Common Illnesses and Injuries

Waking Up Dry: A Guide to Help Children Overcome Bedwetting

Developmental, Behavioral, and Psychosocial Information

Autism Spectrum Disorders: What Every Parent Needs to Know

CyberSafe: Protecting and Empowering Kids in the Digital World of Texting, Gaming, and Social Media

Mental Health, Naturally: The Family Guide to Holistic Care for a Healthy Mind and Body

Immunization Information

Immunizations & Infectious Diseases: An Informed Parent's Guide

Newborns, Infants, and Toddlers

Caring for Your Baby and Young Child: Birth to Age 5*

Dad to Dad: Parenting Like a Pro

Guide to Toilet Training*

Heading Home With Your Newborn: From Birth to Reality

Mommy Calls: Dr. Tanya Answers Parents' Top 101 Questions About Babies and Toddlers

New Mother's Guide to Breastfeeding*

Newborn Intensive Care: What Every Parent Needs to Know

Raising Twins: From Pregnancy to Preschool

Your Baby's First Year*

Nutrition and Fitness

Food Fights: Winning the Nutritional Challenges of Parenthood Armed With Insight, Humor, and a Bottle of Ketchup

A Parent's Guide to Childhood Obesity: A Road Map to Health

Nutrition: What Every Parent Needs to Know

Sports Success R_x! Your Child's Prescription for the Best Experience

School-aged Children and Adolescents

Building Resilience in Children and Teens: Giving Kids Roots and Wings

Caring for Your School-Age Child: Ages 5 to 12

Caring for Your Teenager

Less Stress, More Success: A New Approach to Guiding Your Teen Through College Admissions and Beyond

For more information, please visit the official AAP Web site for parents, www.HealthyChildren.org/bookstore.

*This book is also available in Spanish.

SLEEP

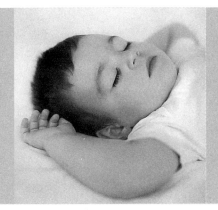

What Every Parent Needs to Know

RACHEL Y. MOON, MD, FAAP

EDITOR IN CHIEF

American Academy of Pediatrics

DEDICATED TO THE HEALTH OF ALL CHILDREN™

Published by the American Academy of Pediatrics
141 Northwest Point Blvd, Elk Grove Village, IL 60007-1019
847/434-4000
Fax: 847/434-8000
www.aap.org

Cover design by Daniel Rembert
Book design by Linda Diamond

Library of Congress Control Number: 2012953639
ISBN: 978-1-58110-781-4

The recommendations in this publication do not indicate an exclusive course of treatment or serve as a standard of medical care. Variations, taking into account individual circumstances, may be appropriate.

The content addressing parent/child scenarios is for information only. The experiences may or may not be suitable for each family and do not indicate an exclusive course of treatment. Before starting any medical treatment or program, you should consult with your child's pediatrician, who can discuss your child's individual needs and counsel you about symptoms and treatment.

Products are mentioned for informational purposes only. Inclusion in this publication does not imply endorsement by the American Academy of Pediatrics. The American Academy of Pediatrics is not responsible for the content of the resources mentioned in this publication. Web site addresses are as current as possible, but may change at any time.

Every effort is made to keep *Sleep: What Every Parent Needs to Know* consistent with the most recent advice and information available from the American Academy of Pediatrics.

CB0073
9-337

1 2 3 4 5 6 7 8 9 10

What People Are Saying

A comprehensive, up-to-date, and useful guide to sleep and sleep disorders in infants, children, and adolescents that will be a valuable go-to resource for parents.

> Judith A. Owens, MD, MPH, FAAP
>
> Director of Sleep Medicine, Children's National Medical Center, and professor of pediatrics, George Washington University School of Medicine and Health Sciences, Washington, DC

Sleep: What Every Parent Needs to Know is a welcome addition to the AAP parent resource library. The basics of sleep and problems that can occur are presented in easy-to-understand language. The format allows parents to easily access just what they need to understand their child's sleep, as well as to find strategies to help with many typical sleep problems of childhood. Tired parents will find help here.

> Debra Babcock, MD
>
> Altos Pediatric Associates

Acknowledgments

Editor

Rachel Y. Moon, MD, FAAP

American Academy of Pediatrics Board of Directors Reviewer

Stuart A. Cohen, MD, MPH, FAAP

Medical Reviewers/Contributors

Debra Ann Babcock, MD, FAAP

Clifford Bloch, MD, FAAP

Nathan J. Blum, MD, FAAP

Waldemar A. Carlo, MD, FAAP

George J. Cohen, MD, FAAP

Olanrewaju Omojokun Falusi, MD

Lori Beth Feldman-Winter, MD, MPH, FAAP

Shelly Vaziri Flais, MD, FAAP

Danette Swanson Glassy, MD, FAAP

Melvin Bernard Heyman, MD, FAAP

Peter B. Kang, MD, FAAP

Paul Kaplowitz, MD, FAAP

Jennifer S. Kim, MD, FAAP

Jane Lynch, MD, FAAP

Juan Carlos Martinez, MD, FAAP, FACCP, DABSM

Camilla Bauman Matthews, MD, FAAP

Judith Anne Owens, MD, FAAP

Stephen J. Pont, MD, MPH, FAAP

Herschel Scher, MD, FAAP

Donald L. Shifrin, MD, FAAP

Benjamin S. Siegel, MD, FAAP

Irene Sills, MD, FAAP

Mary H. Wagner, MD, FAAP

Marc Weissbluth, MD, FAAP

Kupper Wintergerst, MD, FAAP

Manisha B. Witmans, MD, FAAP, FRCPC

Writer

Richard Trubo

From the Editor

To Steve, Sarah, and Elizabeth, with love and gratitude for everything that you've given to me.

To my patients and their families, who have, through the years, been my best teachers.

❧ ❧ ❧ ❧ ❧

Table of Contents

Please Note

The information contained in this book is intended to complement, not substitute for, the advice of your child's pediatrician. Before starting any medical treatment or program, you should consult with your child's pediatrician, who can discuss your child's individual needs and counsel you about symptoms and treatment. If you have questions about how the information in this book applies to your child, speak with your child's pediatrician.

Products mentioned in this book are for informational purposes only. Inclusion in this publication does not constitute or imply a guarantee or an endorsement by the American Academy of Pediatrics.

The information and advice in this book apply equally to children of both sexes (except where noted). To indicate this, we have chosen to alternate between masculine and feminine pronouns throughout the book.

Foreword

The American Academy of Pediatrics (AAP) welcomes you to the latest book in its popular parenting series, *Sleep: What Every Parent Needs to Know.*

Sleep challenges are one of the most common concerns parents and caregivers share with their pediatrician, so it is fitting that the AAP develop a book on this topic. In this book, parents will learn about the ages and stages of sleep, sleep safety, conditions that interfere with your child's sleep, and overall sleep challenges and solutions. This book will also help parents understand how sleep will affect their children as they grow older.

Pediatricians who specialize in sleep and related child health conditions have extensively reviewed this book. Under the direction of its medical editor, the material in this book was developed with the assistance of numerous reviewers and contributors. Because medical information is constantly changing, every effort has been made to ensure that this book contains the most up-to-date findings. Readers may want to visit the AAP Web site for parents, HealthyChildren.org, to keep current on this and other subjects.

It is the hope of the AAP that this book will become an invaluable resource and reference guide to parents. We are confident that parents and caregivers will find the book extremely valuable. We encourage its use along with the advice and counsel of our readers' pediatricians, who will provide individual guidance and assistance related to the health of children.

The AAP is an organization of 60,000 primary care pediatricians, pediatric medical sub-specialists, and pediatric surgical specialists dedicated to the health, safety, and well-being of infants, children, adolescents, and young adults. *Sleep: What Every Parent Needs to Know* is part of ongoing AAP educational efforts to provide parents and caregivers with high-quality information on a broad spectrum of children's health issues.

Errol R. Alden, MD, FAAP
Executive Director/CEO
American Academy of Pediatrics

Introduction

Almost every day in my clinical practice, at least one of my parents brings up a question about sleep. Many parents are unhappy or frustrated because their child isn't sleeping how, when, or where the parents want. Some examples are

"My 2-month-old still isn't sleeping through the night."

"My 3-year-old won't fall asleep until midnight."

"My 7-year-old stays up watching TV until 2:00 in the morning, and then he doesn't want to wake up to go to school."

"My teenager stays awake most of the night and sleeps most of the day on weekends, and then it's so hard to get him up for school."

What I usually find, after a few minutes of asking some questions, is that the sleep problem is often one that could have been avoided. In this book, we offer suggestions for fixing some of these sleep problems—and suggestions for how to avoid some of these sleep problems. As you read through the book, here are some overarching principles that I think may be helpful to consider.

Understand what is "normal" and "typical" for your child's age and stage of development.

I find that a lot of parents overestimate their child's capacity, assuming that a child is just like an adult. For instance, it is virtually impossible for a 2-year-old to sit still for an hour. A 2-year-old is supposed to be zooming around the room, exploring everything, and asking constant questions. That is how she learns about the world. If I have a 2-year-old who sits still without fidgeting or interrupting the parent during even the 5 to 10 minutes that it takes for me to talk to a parent before examining her, I may begin to worry that the child is not developing normally.

Similarly, when I have a parent of a 2-week-old who proudly tells me that her child is "such a good sleeper," sleeping 8 hours at a time, I am concerned because I know that this is not developmentally normal. Babies, until they are about 3 to 5 months old, cannot sleep for more than 5 to 6 hours at a time. (And I consider this time frame "sleeping through the night.") A baby who sleeps longer than that, regardless of what grandparents and neighbors say, is *not* a "good" sleeper. A good sleeper is a baby who awakes frequently but is able to go back to sleep on his own in between feedings every 2 to 4 hours. I often recommend that parents of babies in this age range try to push bedtime back as far as possible so as to allow the baby to sleep until 5:00 or 6:00 am, which is generally more tolerable than if the baby falls asleep at 9:00 pm and awakes at 3:00 am. I remember many nights when my husband or I was walking around our bedroom, holding our baby. Although it was somewhat painful to stay awake until midnight, it was quite nice not to wake up at 3:00 am and realize, with a sinking heart, that sleep for the rest of the night was a lost cause. It was also helpful for us to remember that this was a temporary phase and that things would get better over time.

In addition, all babies and children go through normal developmental phases, which may include nightmares or night terrors. Again, this is normal and typical and will not last forever. Just be patient, and it is likely that this phase will pass after a few months.

All parents want their child to be happy. However, sometimes in an effort to make your child happy in the short term, you can end up creating problems in the long term.

One of my colleagues once said to me, "You are only as happy as your least happy child." This is absolutely true. And I am convinced that every parent, no matter what, wants his child to be happy. You feel sad when your child cries, and you will often do just about anything to keep that from happening. Sometimes, however, this is not good.

I have known parents who have obese children who cannot forgo giving them candy, cookies, and soft drinks because they like to see their child smiling and happy when they are eating. However, they have now created a difficult problem that has long-term consequences. Likewise, I often have parents who want their child to be happy so they put a television or video games in the child's room—or they give a 2-year-old a bottle with milk or juice in it every time she wakes up in the middle of the night. Yes, the child will be happy that evening. But what kind of habits or other long-term consequences (like sleep problems or dental cavities) do those decisions create?

As a parent, you need to think about what will make your child happy in the long run. I am convinced that every child wants to sleep well. And sleeping well is something that you often have to teach your child. It is not something that just "happens." They cannot learn this in school; they cannot learn this from their friends. They can only learn this from their parents. Even though the training process may be painful for a few days, I promise you that it will be worth it in the end.

I once had a parent who came in with her 6-month-old and told me that she and her husband were trying to follow my instructions to get their child to fall asleep on his own. They were going in every 5 to 10 minutes, assuring the baby that they were there and that it was time to go "night-night," and then leaving. The mom burst into tears and said, "Our baby doesn't love me anymore." She thought this because her baby cried even louder every time she left his bedroom. I know the feeling. When we taught both of our children to fall asleep on their own, it was difficult to listen to the crying. I wanted to rescue my child and make her happy again. But somehow I was able to be rational, to keep repeating to myself that "she will thank me in the long run," and after a few nights, all was well. And my daughters still love me.

So take the television out of your child's room. Begin to wean your child off the bottle in the middle of the night. Your child will thank you—maybe not tonight, but in the long run.

Remember who the boss is. In other words, you are stronger than you think you are.

You must remember who the adult—and the boss—is. Children, by nature, are generally not rational beings. You, as the adult, must make the rational decisions and be the boss. I see many families in which the child is the boss. While I will acknowledge that the child is and should be the one who decides when she needs to eat and to have her diaper changed, she is not necessarily the one who is in the best position to decide if she should be in a car seat while traveling or whether or not she should go to school. That is the parent's decision. Similarly, the parent should decide when an appropriate bedtime is; that is not the child's decision. This is often difficult for parents, but you must be strong. A child does not understand and will probably not care that if he stays up watching television until 2:00 am, he will not be happy waking up at 7:00 am and will have a miserable day at school.

Children are very smart, but they need to have consistent rules in their lives to learn what appropriate and inappropriate behavior is. Let's say that you are trying to teach your child how to fall asleep by himself. You have gone in every 10 minutes to check on and reassure your child. After 45 minutes of crying, you are exhausted, decide that you can't take it anymore, and go and pick up your child and bring him into your bed. What have you just taught your child? You have just taught him that if he cries long enough, you will come in and "rescue" him. So what will happen the next night? He will just keep crying for even longer because he has learned that if he cries for long enough, you will eventually come and rescue him again. However, if you remain emotionally strong and resist the temptation to go and pick him up and bring him into your bed, it is most likely that tomorrow night he will cry for a shorter period before falling asleep. And the night after tomorrow he may only cry for 5 minutes before falling asleep. He's learned that you will not rescue him and he has to figure it out himself. That is a good thing for your entire family. But it requires that you be the stronger one. Consistency is the name of the game. You and your partner (or any other adult who cares for your child) must discuss and decide what the rules are going to be. If a child wants to stay up late at night and parents have differing opinions on this matter, the child will fight to stay up, assuming that the parent with the more lenient opinion will win out. This can become a situation in which one parent blames the other and can become quite difficult.

Think about what you want your life to be like in 6 months.

I always ask parents at every checkup where their child sleeps at night. I prefer that a baby sleep in the parents' room for the first 6 to 12 months of the baby's life because room sharing without bed sharing is safest for the baby. If, however, after the baby is 12 months of age, he is still sleeping in the parents' room, I ask, "Is everyone OK with that?" Many times the parents are OK with it but hope that it is a temporary situation. I suggest to parents that they think about what they want the nighttime situation to be in 6 months' time. If they want their child to be sleeping in his own crib or his own room, I suggest that they need to begin working on this now, as it always takes some time to make a change such as this.

You also cannot wait for your child to decide that it is time. You have to decide—and then teach your child how to do it. If your child gets to decide when to give up a pacifier, it may be until she is a teenager (and yes, I have seen teenagers who still use a pacifier at night). Likewise, I have known families in which one or both parents wish for whatever reason that their children slept in a separate bed, but it doesn't happen because they are not proactive about making it happen. (And yes, I've seen families in which teenagers are still sleeping with their parents.) Whatever the scenario, if your child is uncomfortable or unhappy with it—or if one of the adults is uncomfortable or unhappy with it—it needs to be discussed and a decision must be made that everyone can live with.

One of the principal goals of this book is to provide information that is reliable, up-to-date, and evidence-based. *Evidence-based* means that it is based on the evidence—what has been found in research studies. Many experts in pediatric sleep have reviewed this book to ensure that it discusses important topics about pediatric sleep and does so in an evidence-based way. Of course, there are some topics for which there have not been a lot of studies. For these topics I have relied on the consensus of sleep experts. When there is controversy or differing opinions about a particular topic, I have tried to present the pros and cons of each of the opinions and often have presented a "middle ground" approach.

I know that many of you have numerous sources where you get information and advice— besides your pediatrician, you are probably receiving advice from relatives, friends, neighbors, books, magazines, and the Internet. Some of this information can be wildly conflicting, and some of it can be potentially dangerous. You cannot believe everything that people tell you, and you cannot believe everything that you read on the Internet. I hope that this book helps you to navigate the advice you are receiving so that you can make smart decisions that will help your child—and, in turn, your entire family—sleep in a healthier, happier way.

I wish you and your family sweet dreams.

Rachel Y. Moon, MD, FAAP
Editor in Chief

Overview: Basics of Childhood Sleep

Sleep becomes something of an obsession with many new parents. Not only do they worry about whether their baby is getting enough (or too much) sleep, but they also have concerns about their own lack of sleep.

Although medical scientists still do not fully understand all of the functions of sleep, its benefits are obvious. After a good night's sleep, we awake feeling rested, refreshed, and alert. The events we experience during waking hours are integrated into our memory as we sleep. Because sleep gives the body time to repair some of the minor wear-and-tear damage to muscles and other structures, minor aches and pains often disappear during sleep.

Everyone occasionally stays up too late or suffers a sleepless night and then feels groggy and out of sorts the next day. But children who continually fail to get enough sleep do not learn as well as better-rested children. They also have a higher rate of behavior problems. In many cases, overtired children resort to hyperactivity and difficult behavior as a way of fighting off daytime drowsiness.

For parents of newborns or older children with poor sleep habits, the effects of not getting enough sleep can become a constant source of stress. Indeed, new parents often say that a chronic lack of sleep is one of the most trying aspects of adjusting to parenthood.

In the following chapters, you'll find practical advice on how to deal with common sleep problems that can help you and your entire family get a good night's rest. First, however, let's consider some of the basics of sleep.

To Sleep, Perchance to Dream

Virtually every living creature needs to sleep—at least some of the time. And each creature seems to have its own unique sleep pattern. Many of these patterns have evolved over the eons as a response to environmental factors. For example, many creatures share our human preference for sleeping mostly at night when it is dark, quiet, and relatively safe. But night hunters, such as many of the wild cats, sleep mostly during the day and are awake and active at night when their prey is easier to catch. Still others doze off periodically during day and night.

The amount of time spent sleeping also varies greatly. Domestic cats, for example, can sleep 20 or more hours a day, with many short naps interspersed between longer snoozes. Then there are birds, whose sleep includes brief flashes of the kind of nerve activity associated with rapid eye movement (REM) sleep in higher animals (see "Human Stages of Sleep and Sleep Cycles" below). If birds had complete, prolonged REM sleep with its accompanying muscle paralysis, they would topple off their perches. Humans and most other land animals have different stages of sleep, which range from light and partially awake to a state of unconsciousness so deep that it is often described as "dead to the world."

Human Stages of Sleep and Sleep Cycles

Sleep is critical for the development of your child's brain, just as food is important for development of the body. There are 2 basic types of sleep: REM, the "active" sleep when dreams take place, and non-REM, or "quiet" sleep, which is divided into several stages. Each stage is marked by changes in brain waves, muscle activity, eye movements, heart function, and breathing, all of which can be measured by special instruments. Alternating cycles of non-REM and REM sleep make up the sleep stages that occur throughout the night. As we'll point out later, babies have relatively equal amounts of REM versus non-REM sleep during their sleep periods, and they are organized in the following sequence: drowsiness, REM sleep, light sleep, deep sleep, and very deep sleep. (At about 2 to 3 months of age, the pattern will change, cycling through all of the non-REM phases before entering REM sleep.)

Following is a summary of the typical sleep patterns of adults and children by the time they are older than 3 or 4 years.

Non-REM sleep

1. *Stage 1*

   Stage 1 is the brief period (up to 5 minutes) of transition from drowsiness to sleep. Brain activity slows and the eyelids close, although the eyes continue to move together slowly beneath the closed lids. A person is easily awakened, often with a start, from this stage. Sometimes a person may be aware that he is nodding off; at other times, he may think that he is only daydreaming rather than falling asleep.

2. *Stage 2*

   Stage 2 is referred to as light sleep and lasts from 10 to 45 minutes.

3. *Stage 3*

   The deepest state of sleep, stage 3 is characterized by a slowing of brain waves and breathing and heart rate becoming slow and regular. The muscles relax and the child lies very still. He is not easily awakened from stage 3 sleep and if roused, usually takes a minute or so to become fully awake. Stage 3 may last up to 60 minutes. There is then a gradual return to a lighter, stage 2 sleep.

REM Sleep

Occurring after 1 or 2 complete cycles of stages 1 through 3 non-REM sleep, REM sleep is often referred to as active sleep and is the stage during which most dreams occur. The eyes move rapidly under the closed eyelids, breathing and heart rate become less regular, and muscles are more relaxed, although twitching may increase. The first periods of REM sleep of the night usually last for only a few minutes; as the night goes on, however, REM sleep lengthens. This is why many people awaken in the morning while dreaming and may feel as though the entire night has been spent dreaming. Studies in animals and humans suggest that REM sleep is very important; among other things, it keeps the brain active, allows the brain to form memories, and helps the senses develop.

Sleep Cycles

Normal adult sleep is marked by recurring cycles of stages 1 through 3 non-REM sleep, followed by varying periods of REM sleep. Each cycle lasts an average of 90 minutes, although this varies from one person to another and even from one night to another. For example, a person who has gone for several nights without getting enough sleep is likely to spend more time in REM and stage 3 sleep than someone who has been getting adequate sleep.

Influence of Age

As people grow older, sleep patterns and rhythms of biological clocks change (see "Biological Clocks/Circadian Rhythms" on page xxiv). For example, many adolescents experience difficulty falling asleep and prefer to awake late. This is a biologic phenomenon called *delayed*

BIOLOGICAL CLOCKS/CIRCADIAN RHYTHMS

Sleep is one of the many body functions regulated by an inborn biological clock. Medical scientists believe that this clock is centered in 2 tiny clusters of cells deep in the central part of the brain. This biological clock is set according to certain environmental cues, especially periods of daylight and darkness.

The typical human sleep/wake cycle is but one of a number of rhythmic cycles that take about 24 hours to complete; others include a variety of metabolic functions, slight shifts in blood pressure and body temperature, and the secretion of certain hormones. Technically, these 24-hour cycles are referred to as *circadian* (from the Latin meaning "about the day") rhythms. These biological or circadian rhythms are part of our genetic makeup, and they help us stay in sync with the world around us. The body's circadian clock must be set, like a watch, to local time. Travelers who rapidly cross several time zones usually experience jet lag, in which their biological clocks are at odds with the local time. The body automatically resets its clock, but depending upon how many time zones have been crossed, it may take several days to do. Although circadian rhythms are inborn, they take time to develop. This is why young babies have such erratic sleep/wake cycles; initially, these cycles are largely regulated by feelings of hunger or satisfaction (satiety). At about 4 to 6 weeks of age, circadian rhythms begin to develop, starting with hormonal regulation (such as growth hormones and melatonin), and by 8 to 12 weeks, a baby begins to sleep for longer stretches of time; this is called *sleep consolidation and regulation*. At 4 to 6 months of age, most babies are on a regular sleep/wake cycle. It still may not match that of their parents and older siblings, but it pretty much follows a 24-hour pattern.

---

sleep-phase syndrome. It is not merely a result of teenage rebellion but a reflection of altered release of melatonin, the timekeeping hormone (also see Chapter 16, "Melatonin," on page page 204), during puberty and young adulthood.

How a Baby's Sleep Is Different

The sleep of newborns is quite different from that of adults and older children. Before adult-style circadian rhythms develop, newborns typically sleep for 2 or 3 hours at a time, wake up, eat, and soon fall asleep again. They usually sleep for a total of 16 to 18 hours a day, with periods of sleep about equally divided between day and night.

Although many newborns' sleep cycles appear to be random and erratic, the sleep itself follows a pattern, which begins to develop even before birth. Studies indicate that early in the third trimester of gestation, or at about the seventh month of fetal development, babies begin to experience active or REM sleep. A month or so later, quiet or non-REM sleep develops. (At this age, REM and non-REM sleep are called *active* and *quiet* sleep.)

After birth, you can easily tell the difference between the 2 types of sleep. During active sleep, a baby may twitch or flail her arms or legs, and you can see her eyes move under her thin eyelids. Breathing may be somewhat irregular, and she may smile or make sucking motions with her mouth. As in adults, infants' quiet sleep is deeper than their active sleep; breathing is more regular and the baby will not move as much, although she may occasionally twitch or make a sudden movement.

Unlike adults and older children, newborn babies fall directly into active sleep, a pattern that continues until they are about 3 months old. As you've already read, initially sleep is about evenly divided between active and quiet, but this quickly falls to a ratio of 25% active and 75% quiet in an older child or adult. Researchers believe that active sleep plays an important role in brain development, but its exact function is unknown. As the baby grows and her brain becomes more developed, progressively less time is spent in active sleep.

At about 2 months of age, your baby's sleep patterns begin to shift. Sleep becomes more *consolidated,* ie, the baby begins to sleep for longer periods at a time and a preference for nighttime sleep begins to develop. It's important to remember, however, that no 2 babies are exactly alike, and this is certainly true when it comes to sleeping. At 2 months, some babies may sleep for stretches of 5 or 6 hours at night, while others are still waking up and wanting

---

MOTHERS REGULATE CIRCADIAN RHYTHMS IN UNBORN BABIES

Unborn babies are not exposed to light and have no means of telling day from night. Nevertheless, signals from the mother induce the baby to follow the mother's circadian rhythms. The mother's rising and falling levels of melatonin, the timekeeping hormone, pass across the placenta and help to regulate the biological clock in the baby's brain. This helps the baby adjust to regular daily rhythms after birth.

And even though a fetus spends most of its time asleep, an unborn baby is more active while asleep than adults are, which explains why mothers-to-be may feel kicking at all hours of the day and night.

to be fed every 2 or 3 hours. Typically, however, by 2 or 3 months of age, most infants are sleeping for longer periods during the night and staying awake for more of the day, establishing a pattern that carries through until old age, when circadian rhythms may again shift.

PART 1
AGES, STAGES, AND PHASES

All children differ in how much sleep they need, how long it takes them to fall asleep, and how easily they wake up. Many factors influence the quantity and quality of sleep. But because sleep is one of the many body functions regulated by an inborn biological clock, it's important to note that as children grow older, their sleep patterns and rhythms change as well.

CHAPTER 1

The First Year of Life

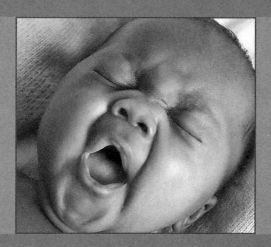

*M*ost parents are prepared for the fact that they will be getting up several times a night once they welcome a new baby into their home. What's surprising for many, when they look back, is how short this period was. For the family's sake, it's important to help young children learn to sleep well because overtired parents and fussy babies are not a happy combination. And while developmentally normal and protective sleep patterns do not necessarily mean more sleep for a baby, good sleep habits will help your children (and the entire family) enjoy their days to the fullest.

It's understandable that so many new parents become obsessed with sleep—not only their own, but also that of their babies. As one mother put it: "When my baby's asleep, I'm constantly checking her to make sure she's breathing and OK. When I'm trying to get some sleep myself, that's when she's wide awake and wants to eat, or be changed, or just have my attention. I now understand the real meaning of sleep deprivation!" Little wonder that a baby's sleeping through the night becomes a major milestone—at least for the parents.

Without any prompting from their parents, newborns get all the sleep they need. When they are not being fed or otherwise tended to, very young babies are likely to be asleep. Undoubtedly, the term *sleeps like a baby* refers to the newborn's innate ability to fall asleep at any time and in any place. But when it comes to parents getting a good night's sleep, the first few weeks of parenthood can be rough indeed.

The journey from helping a newborn fall sleep to when an older baby learns to self-soothe into sleep can take a tremendous emotional as well as physical toll. Some doctors believe that the prolonged depression some new mothers experience is, at least in part, tied to a lack of sleep in the early weeks of caring for a newborn. As the baby begins to sleep for longer periods each night, the depression typically lifts. In any event, chronic lack of sleep can try anyone's patience. It is important for parents to develop strategies that allow them to get enough sleep during the phase when their baby is not yet sleeping through the night. After all, having an "easy" baby is not necessarily what parents want (see "What It *Really* Means to Be a Good Sleeper" on page 12).

IS MY BABY BREATHING NORMALLY?

Healthy babies take from 20 to 60 breaths a minute. Breathing rates are normally quite irregular, and it's not unusual for a baby to pause for up to 20 seconds without taking a breath. This breathing pattern gradually disappears by the time the infant is about 6 months old. It is perfectly normal but can be a heart-stopping event for new parents who are not prepared for it. If your baby stops breathing for longer than 20 seconds, call emergency medical services (911) or your pediatrician.

The Newborn Period

A baby's sleep/wake cycle begins to develop before birth, and by the time the fetus reaches full term, about 60% of his time is spent sleeping or in a sleeplike state. During the first few weeks of life, babies typically sleep most of the time—16 to 20 hours a day. But their sleep is usually in short takes. They sleep for 1 to 4 hours, followed by being awake for 1 to 2 hours. For parents, who are used to doing most of their sleeping in a single stretch at night, this is an adjustment.

Happily, relief is in sight. At 4 weeks of age, most babies begin sleeping for somewhat longer periods during the night, with a longer period of wakefulness during the early evening. Between 4 and 6 weeks of age, sleep begins to consolidate even more in relation to daylight and darkness. In effect, circadian rhythms (see "Biological Clocks/Circadian Rhythms" in the Overview on page xxiv) are being established. For the first 3 months, sleep lasts about 3 to 4 hours. At about 3 to 5 months, healthy babies usually settle into a routine in which they sleep for longer stretches at night—say, 5 to 6 hours—and are awake and active more during the day, with 3 or 4 daytime naps. By 9 months, almost all babies should be able to sleep through the night, or for about 6 to 8 hours, without waking you up. And also by 9 months, most take only 2 daytime naps. There is, however, a big difference between the average and what really happens in any given family. Pediatricians report that issues concerning sleep are near the top of any list of parental concerns.

- "Timmy is now 8 months old, and he still gets us up 2 or 3 times every night. It may take an hour or more to get him back to sleep."

- "Every night it takes me hours to get Shawna settled down enough to stay in bed, and by then I'm totally worn out!"
- "Kelly can't get to sleep unless I'm rocking her. I've tried shutting the door and letting her cry herself to sleep, but after several minutes of listening to her sobbing, I can't stand it anymore, and I end up rocking her for the next hour."

LET SLEEPING BABIES LIE

Healthy, growing babies usually do not need to be awakened to breastfeed or take a bottle. Check with your pediatrician about nighttime awakening if your baby is not doing the following:

- Growing and gaining weight steadily.
- Feeding well 8 to 12 times a day for a breastfeeding baby or 5 to 8 times a day for a bottle-fed baby or older infant.
- Urinating normally with at least 4 wet diapers a day.
- Having at least 3 normal bowel movements per day. Most breastfeeding babies have more frequent bowel movements that are soft and seedy.

The Next Phase

Some babies naturally start to sleep through the night—or at least for a stretch of 3 to 4 hours—when they are 6 to 12 weeks old. More often, however, parents have to give them a bit of a nudge by teaching them to fall asleep on their own. This is important because babies, like older children and adults, go through several periods of arousal and waking during the night. Nobody really "sleeps through the night." When a baby sleeps through the night, it generally means that the baby, when she wakes up in the middle of the night, knows how to comfort herself and goes back to sleep in a few minutes without waking up others. *Babies learn this by being placed in their cribs while still awake.*

Some parents will jump up and move toward their baby when they hear the slightest sound. Many times, the baby is just repositioning or resettling himself. Give him a few minutes to go back to sleep on his own before you make a move. Even if he begins to wail, resist attending to him for a few minutes. If the crying continues, go to the crib and pat him gently in a soothing manner to see if that will calm him down enough for him to settle back down

SWADDLING CAN HELP A BABY SLEEP

My 6-week-old thrashes about and cries out when she sleeps. She continually hits herself in the face and wakes up. Is this behavior normal? How do I help her to sleep better?

Many babies move about and whimper in their sleep. They sometimes wake themselves because they cannot yet control the movements of their hands and arms. This is normal.

One way to help comfort your baby until she has better motor control (about 2 months) is by *swaddling*—that is, wrap her from the shoulders down in a sheet or lightweight receiving blanket. Some babies sleep well if they are swaddled firmly; others seem to prefer a lighter wrap that lets them keep their arms partly free. Some babies like their arms swaddled; others are more comfortable when their arms are outside the swaddle. You want to make sure that you don't swaddle your baby too tightly, as this can make it more difficult for her to breathe or can cause problems with her hips. As your baby develops more motor control, she will need less swaddling. Once your baby is 2 months old, swaddling is not recommended because she may roll onto her side or stomach while swaddled and not be able to roll back onto her back. If you swaddle your baby, make sure that she is always placed on the back while she is swaddled. Never place a swaddled baby on the side or stomach. Keep an eye on the swaddled baby to make sure she hasn't rolled onto her side or stomach.

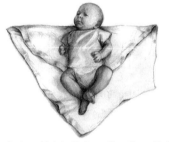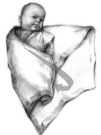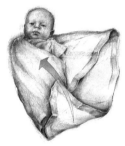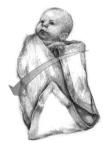

1. Lay a thin baby blanket out like a diamond in front of you.
2. Fold the top corner of the blanket down a bit so that the folded corner almost reaches the middle of the blanket.
3. Place your infant on his back, centered on the blanket with his arms at his sides and his head just above the folded edge and his shoulders just below it.
4. Take one of the side corners of the blanket and fold it over your baby's shoulder and across his body, making sure to tuck the corner underneath him on the opposite side.
5. Then take the bottom corner of the blanket (below your baby's feet) and fold it up over your baby. If the blanket is large enough that the bottom corner reaches up to (or over) your baby's face, you can simply fold it back down until his face is no longer covered or bring it over either shoulder and tuck it under him.
6. Finally, take the only remaining corner and pull it over your baby's other shoulder and across his body. Again, tuck this corner snugly under your baby's opposite side.

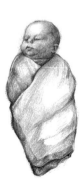

on his own. If you need to pick him up and feed him, change his diaper, or other things, do them quickly without fuss and without making it playtime. You want to send a message that it's sleep time, not playtime. Place him back in his crib while he's drowsy but still not entirely asleep. This consistent approach will help your baby learn to fall asleep on his own in his crib.

There are some concrete ways to help your newborn learn how to sleep.

- Help him fall asleep with a soothing sensation, such as rocking, sucking a thumb or hand, or nonnutritive suckling at the breast. However, never place your baby in the crib with a bottle for comfort. The natural sugar in many liquids promotes growth of the bacteria that cause tooth decay, and the effect is especially severe when the sugary residue stays in the mouth all night long. This can result in serious dental decay, known as *nursing bottle caries,* in developing primary teeth. Liquid, even water, pooling in the mouth can also back up through the *eustachian tubes,* the tiny passages that run between the throat and ear. This can set up conditions that foster the development of ear infections.
- Give him lots of attention while he is awake. Especially early on, babies need help to feel calm and secure. Holding your baby and being sensitive to his signals and needs will not spoil him or reinforce a behavior.
- Pay attention to signs of being sleepy or overtired. By noticing your baby's cues early on you'll also have an opportunity to help him fall asleep before he is overtired. These signs will become easier to identify as you get to know your baby, and in turn, it will become easier for you to settle him for sleep.

The bottom line is to meet your baby's needs early on so that he will be better able to regulate his sleep cycles and emotions.

GOOD NIGHT, MOON...

Even as early as 6 to 8 weeks you can establish a predictable bedtime routine: washing up, changing into sleepwear, a few minutes "reading" a picture book, a gentle song, saying good night to toys or pictures in the room. Activities performed in the same order each night make up a soothing ritual that helps put your baby in the mood for sleep.

Stages of Newborn Sleep

Sleep patterns in newborns are different from those in older children and adults. For newborns, sleep is about equally divided between rapid eye movement (REM) and non-REM sleep and follows these stages:

Stage 1: Drowsiness, in which the baby starts to fall asleep.

Stage 2: REM sleep (also referred to as *active sleep),* in which the baby may twitch or jerk her arms or legs, and her eyes move under her closed eyelids. Breathing is often irregular and may stop for 5 to 10 seconds—a condition called *normal periodic breathing of infancy*—then start again with a burst of rapid breathing at the rate of 50 to 60 breaths a minute for 10 to 15 seconds, followed by regular breathing until the cycle repeats itself. The baby's skin color does not change with the pauses in breathing and there is no cause for concern (in contrast with apnea; see Chapter 12, Sleep Apnea, pages 171–177). Babies generally outgrow periodic breathing by about the middle of the first year.

Stage 3: Light sleep, in which breathing becomes more regular and sleep becomes less active.

Stages 4 and 5: Deep non-REM sleep (also referred to as *quiet sleep).* Twitching and other movements cease, and the baby falls into sleep that becomes progressively deeper. During these stages, the baby may be more difficult to awake.

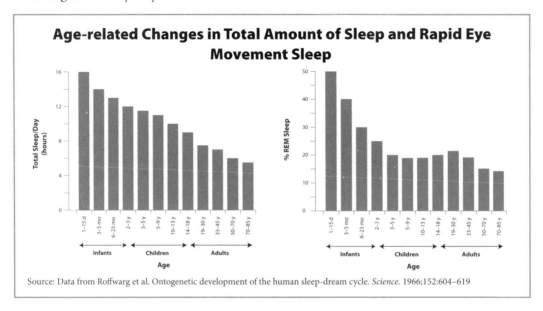

Age-related Changes in Total Amount of Sleep and Rapid Eye Movement Sleep

Source: Data from Roffwarg et al. Ontogenetic development of the human sleep-dream cycle. *Science.* 1966;152:604–619

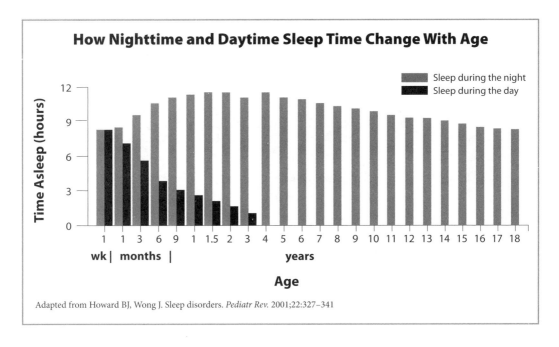

How Nighttime and Daytime Sleep Time Change With Age

Adapted from Howard BJ, Wong J. Sleep disorders. *Pediatr Rev.* 2001;22:327–341

The First 6 Months

Most newborns are sleeping or drowsy for 16 to 20 hours a day. Some wake at fairly regular 2-hour intervals, whereas others may occasionally sleep as long as 4 or 6 hours at a stretch. It's difficult to place newborns on a strict schedule because their internal clocks are not yet functioning. At about 6 weeks, the daily cycles we call circadian rhythms (see "Biological Clocks/Circadian Rhythms" in the Overview on page xxiv) start to become established.

By about 16 weeks, many babies are adapting to a light/dark schedule. They sleep more at night and remain alert for increasingly longer periods in the daytime. This rhythm comes about, in part, thanks to behavioral cues from parents and caregivers, who encourage their baby to play more during daytime waking periods. By contrast, nighttime waking should be kept calm, quiet, and no longer than necessary to change, feed, and burp baby and return him—comfortable, sleepy, but still awake—to his crib or bassinet. (For detailed information about the right way to position your baby for sleep, see Chapter 2, Babies and Sleep Safety, pages 29–30.)

Even as babies become more alert and playful, many continue to take 2 or more daytime naps for at least the first 6 months. The morning nap gradually drops out, but for most children, the afternoon nap continues through toddlerhood and into the preschool years. If, after the first few weeks, your baby is constantly drowsy, sleeps most of the time, and never seems fully awake, consult your pediatrician.

WHAT IT *REALLY* MEANS TO BE A GOOD SLEEPER

It's important for parents, caregivers, families, and friends to understand that at this age, a good sleeper is a child who wakes up frequently but can get himself back to sleep. It is *not* a child who sleeps without waking for 10 hours at night. Frequent waking is developmentally appropriate and allows the baby to wake up when he is in a situation in which he is not getting enough oxygen or is having problems breathing. Sleeping undisturbed for prolonged periods at this age is not healthy.

Granted, some lucky parents escape such traps. Between the ages of 3 and 6 months, their babies naturally seem to fall into a happy routine: They go to bed with hardly a whimper, sleep for 5 to 7 hours at a stretch during the night, and take a couple of lengthy naps during the day. When they are awake, they are cheerful and alert. Of course, there may be restless nights when their baby is fussy or sick, but these are the exception rather than the rule, and the baby soon returns to his normal routine.

For all too many parents, however, this sounds like an impossible dream. But it doesn't need to be that way. Good sleep habits can be encouraged almost from the very beginning. You may need to experiment a bit, but in general, here's how to begin, even before your baby is ready to sleep for more than a few hours at a time.

1. Start by helping *set the sleep/wake cycle of your baby's inborn biological clock.* This internal clock takes important cues from the outside world. Your goal is to have the sleep cycle coincide with nighttime. Many new mothers insist that rooming-in at the hospital, in which they keep their babies in their own quiet, darkened room at night rather than in a brightly lit hospital nursery, even though it's only for a night or two, makes a difference. If rooming-in is not possible, you can start the readjustment as soon as you take your baby home. During the day, open the blinds to let daylight in or turn on the lights in the baby's room, even when he is sleeping.

THE IMPORTANCE OF SLEEP ASSOCIATIONS

Sleep associations are important for all of us. These are the conditions that you are used to having when falling asleep, and so these are the conditions that you need to have present before you can fall back to sleep in the middle of the night. Many adults have a sleep association with a pillow. If, in the middle of the night, you wake up and cannot find your pillow, you cannot go back to sleep until you have found that pillow again and placed it right where you are used to having it when you fall asleep.

Babies and children develop sleep associations as well. Some common sleep associations are
- Being rocked to sleep
- Sucking a pacifier or finger
- Suckling at the breast
- Drinking a bottle of formula
- Having the television on while falling asleep

As you can see, some of these sleep associations may pose a problem in the middle of the night if your baby wakes up. If her sleep association is being rocked to sleep, she will not be able to go back to sleep in the middle of the night unless you get up and rock her back to sleep.

It is important for babies and children to form sleep associations that make it easy for them to fall back asleep by themselves in the middle of the night. We therefore recommend that babies be placed in their cribs while drowsy but still awake. This creates a positive sleep association with the feeling of being in the crib.

---

2. *Expose your baby to normal levels of daytime noise.* Don't feel you have to whisper and tiptoe around. When a baby is tired, he'll sleep through a normal amount of noise. But if he becomes used to a super-quiet environment, he may become overly sensitive to noise, and every little nighttime sound will awaken him.

3. *During the day, encourage your baby to stay awake for longer periods.* Use this time to cuddle, play with, and get to know your baby. This is a great opportunity for tummy time (see "Tummy Time: A Primer" on page 31). If your baby spends most of the day sleeping and is awake most of the night, try to reverse the pattern by waking him to eat and play during the day.

4. *As evening approaches, switch to a dimmer and quieter environment.* Spend less time playing and giving extra attention. Place your baby for sleep in a darkened, quiet room. Your baby is still likely to wake up every 2 or 3 hours, but given the right environmental cues, this should begin to change in a few weeks. Your baby will be more awake and active during the day, and nighttime sleep periods will become a bit longer. By 6 to 8 weeks of age, some babies start skipping one of the nighttime feedings.

A newborn often falls fast asleep while feeding or being rocked and does not wake up when being put in bed. But after the newborn phase—at about 6 to 8 weeks of age—it's time for your baby to start learning how to go to sleep on his own. Don't rock a baby to sleep or allow him to doze off while feeding. Sing or talk to your baby in a soft voice, stroke his head, and play with his feet. Let him get groggy or drowsy, and then place him on his back in his crib while he is still drowsy but before he is fully asleep. At first, he may become more awake and fuss or even cry. Draw the shades or turn down the lights; tell him good night in a soft, loving voice; and go to your bed.

SLEEP PATTERNS IN A PREMATURE BABY

My son is now 17 weeks old; however, he was a preemie and is only 8 weeks according to his corrected age. He only sleeps through the night on rare occasions and his sleep patterns are erratic. Will they settle down soon?

Premature babies tend to wake more often at night than full-term babies, at least for the first several months. Night waking and lighter sleep are part of a survival and developmental mechanism that protects preemies. Their systems for breathing and circulation are under the control of a nervous system that is not yet mature. This keeps a premature baby in a state in which he is more easily aroused for feeding. Preemies spend more of their sleep time in rapid eye movement sleep, and child development specialists believe that this may be part of a mechanism that helps the brain develop normally. Your baby will settle in time, but you should be prepared for frequent night waking during the next few months.

Waking During the Night

Some 3- or 4-month-old babies will be able to sleep for a long stretch—say 5 or 6 hours—during the night. But others may wake up every couple of hours. Don't rush to the crib every time you hear your baby whimper—wait a few minutes and see if she'll fall back asleep without attention. But if your baby's cry is one of distress or it persists for more than a few minutes, by all means go to her.

BREAST AND BOTTLE

My sister's baby, who is bottle-fed, started sleeping through the night when he was barely 3 months old. My breastfed baby is 2 months older and still wants to be fed 2 or 3 times during the night. My sister says breastfed babies are slower to sleep through the night than those who are bottle-fed. Is this true?

While breastfed babies initially awaken more during the night for feedings and feed more times per day, their sleep patterns—falling asleep, staying asleep, and total sleep time—stabilize in later infancy and are similar to sleep patterns in non-breastfed babies by 6 months of age.

However, breastfed babies generally do want more frequent feedings, including during the night, for a longer period than babies who are fed formula. Some experts attribute this to the fact that human milk is easier and faster to digest than formula. Thus, a meal of human milk may be digested in 2 or 3 hours, and the baby will be ready to feed again. Also, breastfed babies who are used to falling asleep while on the breast may have difficulty getting back to sleep unless they are allowed to nurse. To encourage your baby to start sleeping through the night, try changing your nighttime responses. Don't rush in at the first whimper; instead, wait a few minutes to see if your baby will fall back to sleep. And don't let her fall asleep while nursing. Instead, put her in the crib drowsy but awake and let her fall asleep on her own. Any sleep difficulties associated with breastfeeding will resolve over time, especially if you address troublesome sleep associations.

Avoid turning on the light if possible. Check whether she needs changing; if so, try to change the diaper without picking your baby up. After she calms down, say good night in a soft voice and leave the room. A baby who has learned to put herself to sleep will probably doze off in a few minutes.

THE SOLID FOOD MYTH

My baby is almost 3 months old and still wakes up at least once or twice during the night. My mother insists that I could solve the problem by giving him some cereal in the evening. However, my pediatrician says to wait. Who's right?

Follow your pediatrician's advice. The American Academy of Pediatrics recommends waiting until about 6 months of age before introducing solid foods. There's no relationship between starting solid foods and sleeping through the night. Many babies start sleeping through the night before starting solid foods, while others still want a nighttime feeding even though they are eating solid foods during the day. At 3 months of age, your baby needs the extra calories and nutrition provided by human milk or formula.

WHERE WE STAND

The American Academy of Pediatrics recommends exclusive breastfeeding for the first 6 months of life and that mothers continue breastfeeding for at least 12 months or as long as baby and mother want to continue.

The Question of Crying

Typically, newborns and young babies cry an average of 2½ to 3 hours a day. While it's normal for babies to cry, it's also normal for parents to want the crying to stop. But it's important to realize that crying is a baby's major means of communication and that not every cry is a sign of hunger or distress. Granted, babies cry when they are hungry, in pain, or need changing, but they also cry when they are bored, overstimulated, annoyed, or simply need attention. It doesn't take parents long to be able to interpret their baby's cries and to respond appropriately.

Colic is another matter. Without a doubt, parents find infant colic one of the most frustrating and difficult forms of crying, because the crying is not something that the parents can "fix." Typically, the crying occurs at about the same time on most days, usually in the late afternoon or evening, and lasts for 3 or more hours at a time. The baby may pass gas or draw up his legs as if in pain. After several hours of wailing, the crying stops as abruptly as it began and the baby falls into a peaceful sleep. By that time, however, the parents are distraught, nervous wrecks.

Usually, the baby's pediatrician cannot find a physical cause for the crying. A number of theories as to what causes colic have been advanced—for example, allergies, an immature gastrointestinal system, overstimulation—but none have been proved. It's likely that a combination of factors is involved. Some experts say that in certain babies, colic may be a variation of normal behavior. Babies typically cry for 2½ to 3 hours over the course of a day, but a colicky baby may be doing all his crying at one stretch. In any event, about 1 in 5 babies develop colic. Difficult as colic is, parents can take comfort in the fact that it rarely lasts beyond 4 or 5 months of age.

Special Situations

Breastfed babies typically start sleeping through the night somewhat later than babies who are bottle-fed, and they may need a nighttime feeding for longer. But it may help to remember that breastfeeding provides many health benefits to your baby, including increased immunity against diseases in the first year of life and a reduced risk of sudden infant death syndrome. And remember that by age 5 or 6 months, breastfed babies should sleep 6 to 7 hours at a time during the night (see "Breast and Bottle" on page 15).

Premature babies also take longer to sleep through the night. In general, a baby who was born prematurely needs extra time to sleep through the night; the amount of extra time is generally the number of weeks early he was born. For example, a baby who is born 6 weeks before term may take an extra 6 or 7 weeks to reach this milestone. Although it may take longer to achieve the ultimate goal, you still should work on instilling good sleep habits by placing the baby in his crib while he is still awake and helping him learn to go to sleep on his own.

AN INFANT WHO WON'T LIE DOWN

My 8-month-old gets so tired that he falls asleep sitting up in his crib. How can I get him to lie down before he falls asleep?

You don't have to force your baby to lie down. By now he has good enough motor control that after tumbling to the mattress, he can find a comfortable position for himself and sleep soundly the rest of the night.

However, more interrupted nights are probably in store with the appearance of separation anxiety during the second half of the first year. Somewhere between 6 and 12 months, your infant, who used to be outgoing and friendly even with people he didn't know, may start to become tense and fearful when strangers come too close. He may even get upset at the sight of family members or regular babysitters, especially if they approach abruptly. At the same time, he'll cling when you have to leave him or pass him to someone else to hold. If he finds himself in unfamiliar surroundings, he may appear uneasy and look to you for reassurance. This is separation anxiety, a normal phase and an important step forward in your child's emotional development. It indicates that your baby is becoming aware of himself as an individual separate from you. He is also beginning to understand that you too are a separate person.

Separation anxiety generally peaks between 10 and 18 months of age and gradually fades away during the latter half of the second year. Babies in this period often call out or cry for their parents in the middle of the night. Sometimes they are able to pull themselves up to stand in their cribs but can't get back down. They may need help to reposition themselves for sleep. Keep interactions with your child loving, supportive, brief, and matter-of-fact. Check with your pediatrician for additional strategies to reduce the duration of this phase. (For more about separation anxiety, see "Night Waking" on page 21.)

SECURITY BLANKETS = STRESS BUSTERS

The period between 8 and 15 months is usually the time when children become attached to transitional objects, cuddly blankets, toys, or sometimes unusual choices that help them make the emotional passage from dependence to independence. Having a comforting, familiar transitional object helps your child feel at home in a strange place, reassures him when he's away from you, calms him when he's upset, and helps him relax into sleep. It's a good idea to help your child blend a transitional object into his bedtime ritual by keeping a small, cuddly blanket or very small, soft toy in the crib. However, to prevent the possibility of accidental suffocation, soft transitional objects, such as pillows, blankets, cushions, or stuffed toys, should not be placed in the crib with your child until he is at least 1 year old.

For many children, a pacifier is the favored transitional object, and this is especially appropriate in the first 6 months of life. The American Academy of Pediatrics suggests that a pacifier can be offered, once breastfeeding has been well-established, at bedtime up to the age of 6 to 12 months. Not only does this provide a transitional object, but it may reduce the risk of sudden infant death syndrome as well. Some people worry that pacifier use may make it more likely for a baby to get ear infections, but this usually doesn't happen until 6 to 12 months of age. Language begins to develop at about 6 months, and some pediatricians would recommend that you try to limit the pacifier to bedtime use only at this point or to begin to wean the pacifier altogether because a child with a pacifier constantly in his mouth at that time may not babble and speak as much as other children.

If the transitional object also becomes an indispensable daytime companion, as many do, you may want to keep a duplicate so you can wash and dry one while the other is on duty. A transitional object is a stress buster that the child will gradually give up on his own as he finds more mature ways to deal with life's challenges.

During the separation anxiety phase, your baby may also become fearful around objects and situations he used to take for granted. For example, his nighttime waking may be complicated by fear of the dark, or he may be frightened by loud noises or a thunderstorm. A night-light in the bedroom helps to banish fear of the dark. And although you may often have to go into your child's bedroom to reassure him with calming words or a gentle back rub, at other times he may settle back to sleep after you call out to let him know you're in the next room or on your way to comfort him.

SLEEP AND GROWTH HORMONE

Growth is dependent on the interplay of several hormones. The main one is growth hormone, which is secreted by the pituitary gland. Although growth hormone is secreted during the day, the highest blood levels occur while children are sleeping at night. All children need adequate sleep to grow properly, and at every age children need more sleep than adults. Children need extra sleep during the massive growth spurts that take place during infancy and adolescence. It does not follow, however, that a child's growth will be stunted if she sleeps less than others her age or that a child who sleeps a lot will be tall. Children's height is programmed in the genes they inherit. What's important, therefore, is that each child gets as much sleep as she needs to keep up a satisfactory rate of growth and a good level of activity.

Night Waking in the First Year

Somewhere around the middle of the first year, babies mature to a point where they can get through 5 to 7 hours at night without a feeding and can soothe themselves back to sleep when they awaken but are not hungry or uncomfortable for some other reason.

If your baby wakes up and cries in obvious distress, attend to her needs promptly and gently, without a fuss. When your baby is calm and drowsy but still awake, put her back in her crib and say good night. If your baby whimpers, give her a few minutes to settle on her own. If the crying shows no sign of letting up and you can hear your baby becoming distressed, return briefly to comfort her. She may be feeling the first stirrings of separation anxiety and may need a little reassurance that you are nearby. Keep the room dim, try gently patting or rubbing her, but avoid picking her up if you can. When she is calm, return to your bed again. Repeat the procedure, if necessary, at increasingly longer intervals but no more than about 10 minutes, until your baby settles back to sleep.

Six to 12 Months

By the time your baby is 6 months old, you may expect him to sleep for 13 to 15 hours a day, with 60% to 70% of these sleeping hours during the night. For some lucky parents, these hours will occasionally take place in a single stretch. At this age, babies are wide awake and active during play periods and usually sleep well after interludes of intense activity. Between

6 and 10 months babies typically try to pull themselves upright on furniture and in their cribs. They tire themselves out with the intense physical effort and concentration needed to master these and other complex movements, such as rolling over, reaching, and attempting to become mobile while crawling. This allows them to sleep for longer periods at night. But remember, no 2 babies are exactly alike, especially when it comes to establishing a sleep/wake schedule. Some are sleeping for 5 to 7 hours during the night at 6 weeks; others don't reach this landmark until 6 months.

FREQUENT WAKING AT 6 MONTHS

If your 6-month-old baby regularly wakes up several times during the night, bring it to your pediatrician's attention. Your pediatrician can check your baby to make sure that there is nothing wrong. In addition, your pediatrician can provide suggestions for how to get your baby to sleep for longer periods at night. (See also Chapter 3.)

NIGHT WAKING

My 9-month-old baby used to sleep all night, but suddenly, without any reason, he is waking in the middle of the night. His teeth don't seem to be bothering him, he hasn't been sick, and he is growing and developing well. What could be the cause?

Waking phases come and go, often without any explanation, in the first few years. As long as your baby is healthy, well fed, and comfortable (bedroom not too warm or cold, diaper not soaked and clammy), this may be just a stage in his development. It may also be that your baby is experiencing the onset of *separation anxiety,* a normal developmental stage in which the child fears the loss of his primary caregiver and becomes wary of unfamiliar faces. During this period, infants and toddlers often wake once or many times in the night and may even call for one parent in preference to the other.

When your baby cries, give him a few minutes to settle down on his own. If the crying continues, keep the lights dim as you check to make sure everything is all right, pat your baby and reassure him but avoid picking him up, and leave his room again as soon as he is calm but still awake. During the daytime, play lots of variations on peekaboo to help your baby anticipate your return.

For more about separation anxiety, see pages 18 and 19.

No Time to Sleep

Infants are often wakeful at night around the time they reach major milestones. They may also seem impatient and irritable during the daytime. It's as if the baby is so eager to master a new skill, be it standing up or walking alone, that she can't stop doing it and certainly can't be bothered with routine activities such as eating, dressing, and sleeping.

For example, an infant who has just learned how to stand in her crib may not yet know how to sit back down. Something like this may prolong night waking. Unless she doesn't mind tumbling to the mattress, she may call her parents over and over to help her down, only to repeat the performance minutes later. You can teach your new Homo erectus to get down by gently supporting her while pressing firmly against the backs of her knees until they buckle. Practice this maneuver during the day. Your baby will soon get the hang of it. When she does, she will again be able to relax and settle for sleep or go on to a new phase—perhaps babbling her newest sounds or getting ready to walk alone.

PARENTS MAY PROJECT THEIR OWN FEELINGS ONTO CRYING BABIES

Psychologists who have studied the behavior of thousands of children caution parents not to over-interpret babies' crying. An older child can explain her feelings. But parents don't always know why a young baby cries. What they hear, therefore, may reflect their own moods and concerns rather than their baby's wants. A baby who cries just after being put into her crib may be only letting off steam. She's not necessarily saying, "I'm lonely," or "You're cruel to abandon me," or even "You'll have to listen to this crying forever." Resist the urge to rush back and rescue her. Your baby may just feel like vocalizing before she settles down to sleep.

Parents Need Sleep Too

Try not to feel let down when you're still waking frequently even after your baby starts sleeping through the night. The reason is that your body needs time to readjust and settle back into its former sleeping patterns. However, if you had sleep troubles before your baby came on the scene, it's likely that the same problems will reappear or continue.

Lack of sleep affects every aspect of our functioning—not least, the way we function as parents. When we get enough sleep, we tend to be happier and less anxious and depressed; our memory is better and we perform job-related duties better. Fatigue due to lack of sleep is a leading cause of road crashes, causing injuries and fatalities everywhere in the world.

Adults need on average 8 hours of sleep a night. Some get by on about 7, while others perform best after 9 or 10 hours. Those who get less than 7 hours, however, are almost always sleep deprived. People who are sleep deprived look and feel washed out and tend to get drowsy at odd times throughout the day. Evaluated under laboratory conditions, their sleep patterns differ according to whether they are sleep deprived or well rested.

Sleep is important throughout life, and not only when your child is a baby. If tasks are keeping you up past your bedtime, try to deal with the most pressing ones and schedule the others at times that won't interfere with your rest. Perhaps you could delegate some of the chores at a modest cost. Or your older children may be mature enough to take on regular chores and possibly to trade extra help for an allowance. If naps refresh you (some people feel groggy rather than well-rested after a nap), time regular naps to fit in with your child's schedule. Breastfeeding mothers often find it easier to take advantage of naps when their babies are sleeping, as hormones secreted during breastfeeding naturally make you sleepy. Take care that naps don't interfere with your nighttime sleep. If you usually have trouble falling asleep or have an irregular sleep/wake cycle, naps may not be a solution for you.

Keep to a regular schedule for going to bed and waking up, even on weekends. Sleeping late on weekends doesn't make up for sleep lost during the week. Avoid caffeine, if it keeps you awake, and alcohol, which may make you sleepy at first but can cause wakefulness later in the night. Ask your physician's advice about sleep problems.

Many commonly used medications are known to influence the quality and quantity of our sleep. They include antidepressants, antihistamines, decongestants, and cough and cold remedies. Some women are surprised to find that sleep troubles disappear when they switch from oral contraceptive pills to other forms of birth control. Even sleeping pills, muscle relaxants, and sedatives can cause sleep difficulties. Although such medications may originally have been prescribed for reasons unrelated to sleep, eventually the body comes to depend on them and, in time, the user finds it difficult to get to sleep without them. Avoid nonprescription sleeping remedies, which can have a rebound effect and make your sleep troubles worse.

Sleep experts caution that any substance that affects the nervous system is likely to have an effect on our sleep. Nicotine, a stimulant drug, is one example. Even though you may be a nonsmoker, smoke from others' cigarettes may make it hard for you to get to sleep after a social event and leave you feeling poorly rested and hungover the next morning.

Anxiety and depression commonly interfere with sleep in 2 ways. In a depressed or anxious state we may find it difficult to fall asleep, or we may wake up with a start and remain wide-eyed and anxious through the early morning hours. Either way, the anxious person doesn't sleep enough, feels exhausted during the day, and may face each succeeding night with increasing anxiety about not getting the sleep he needs. And although insomnia often occurs with emotional upset, depression can also lead a person to sleep many more hours than usual and wake up feeling groggy, tired—and still depressed.

If you have physical or emotional problems that are interfering with your sleep—or even if you don't have any problems and you still can't sleep—schedule an appointment with your doctor, who will be able to suggest behavioral and lifestyle measures. When sleep troubles are deep-seated, your doctor may recommend consultation with another specialist.

SWITCH TO "BABY TIME"

As much as possible, go on "baby time" for the first few months. Catch a nap when your baby is sleeping and for the time being, forget about trying to do all your sleeping in a single nighttime stretch. Save your energy for getting to know and enjoying your new baby.

You may be lucky enough to have help to pitch in with laundry, housework, and other chores. If not, perhaps you could work out a system with other new parents in your neighborhood, trading off babysitting, food shopping, and household tasks. In this way, each member of the "cooperative" could count on an uninterrupted stretch 2 or 3 times a week for napping or catching up on chores. Another possibility might be to hire a high school or college student as a helper for a few hours each week.

Consistency, Consistency

Babies are fast learners, especially when it comes to getting their parents to respond to their wishes. Of course, you should heed your baby's demands for food, changing, and attention. And you should take time to cuddle—and savor getting to know—this marvelous little person. At the same time, you must help your baby learn good sleep habits as a prelude to other steps in self-discipline and self-reliance. This requires a consistent approach and establishing a set bedtime routine (see Chapter 5).

Remember too that there are no absolute rules that work for everyone; common sense must prevail. Find what seems to work best for you and your baby, and then stick to it. If your baby is teething or has a cold, you may need to alter bedtime and nap-time routines until the situation goes back to normal. A baby who is sick needs extra cuddling, care, and attention until her symptoms clear up and she feels well again. But then return to the established routine. This way, the entire family can enjoy a good night's sleep!

CHAPTER 2

Babies and Sleep Safety

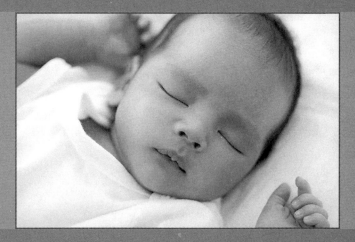

*F*ew things are as comforting to parents as watching their baby sleeping peacefully. At the same time, however, a baby's sleep time is often not anxiety-free. It may bring to mind the term sudden infant death syndrome, *or SIDS, leading some moms and dads to wonder whether they have done everything possible to keep their baby safe during sleep. True, there has been a major decrease in the incidence of SIDS; but even so, SIDS remains responsible for more infant deaths in the United States than any other cause during the first year of life (beyond the newborn period). In addition, there are accidental deaths, such as suffocation or strangulation, that can occur while baby is sleeping.*

Fortunately, there are steps you can take to help reduce your own baby's risk of SIDS and other potential problems related to her sleep environment. These guidelines for safe sleep should be shared with everyone who cares for your baby.

Reducing the Risk of Sudden Infant Death Syndrome and Accidental Sleep-Related Deaths

Sudden infant death syndrome is the unexpected and sudden death of a child younger than 1 year for which no explainable cause is found. Theories about the cause of SIDS range from infections and milk allergies to soft bedding and stuffed toys. None, however, has been proven to be the single cause; in all probability, multiple factors play a role. About 3 decades ago, pediatricians in several countries, including the United States, discovered that the number of deaths from SIDS can be reduced by up to half when babies are *not* placed on the side or stomach to sleep. So since 1992, when a "back to sleep" recommendation was introduced, deaths from SIDS have decreased from more than 5,000 per year to the current figure of less than 2,500 per year.

So unless your doctor has advised otherwise, always place your baby to sleep on her back. Side sleeping is not safe and is not advised. Despite what some people believe, sleeping on the back *does not* increase a baby's risk of choking. In fact, babies who sleep on their backs are less likely to choke or aspirate. This is because when babies are on their backs, if food comes up the esophagus, it has to go up against gravity to go into the trachea and lungs (which is what aspiration is). Anatomically, it is more difficult to aspirate on the back as opposed to on the stomach. (See illustration below.) This is the case even for those babies with gastro-esophageal reflux or GER (spitting up stomach contents) because they have protective airway mechanisms. The American Academy of Pediatrics (AAP) and the North American Society for Pediatric Gastroenterology, Hepatology and Nutrition recommend that babies with GER should sleep on their backs unless there is an anatomic or neurologic reason that the airway is not protected against aspiration (for instance, by a normal gag reflex).

Baby Upper Respiratory Anatomy

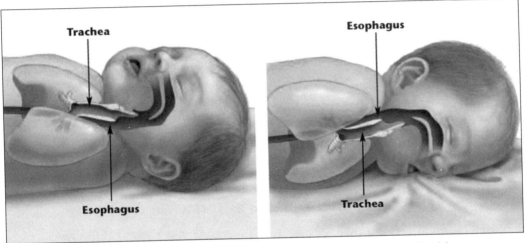

Baby in the Back-Sleeping Position   **Baby in the Stomach-Sleeping Position**

Source: US Department of Health and Human Services. National Institute of Child Health and Human Development. *Continuing Education Program on SIDS Risk Reduction.* December 2006

It's also important not to elevate the head of your baby's crib when she's in it and on her back. Not only is it ineffective for reducing GER, but she may slide to the foot of the crib, which may jeopardize her ability to breathe.

While it's important to position your baby on her back for sleep, she should have plenty of tummy time down on the floor when she is awake and being watched. This is necessary to help her strengthen her upper body and arms and develop her motor skills.

TUMMY TIME: A PRIMER

Tummy time is for babies who are awake and being watched. Your baby needs this to develop strong muscles. It also helps to prevent skull flattening, which can sometimes happen if a baby spends too much awake time on her back.

Beginning on the first day home from the hospital or in your family child care home or center, play and interact with your baby while he is awake and on his tummy 2 to 3 times each day for a short time (3–5 minutes), increasing the amount of time as your baby shows he enjoys the activity. A great time to do this is following a diaper change or when your baby wakes up from a nap. If your baby is going to day care, ask your child care provider to provide some tummy time.

Tummy time prepares babies for the time when they will be able to slide on their bellies and crawl. As babies grow older and stronger they will need more time on their tummies to build their own strength.

What if my baby does not like being on her tummy?

Some babies may not like the tummy time position at first. Place yourself or a toy in reach for her to play with. You may be tempted to end tummy time quickly if your baby doesn't seem happy. Resist that urge! Start with at least 3 minutes (set a timer, if that will strengthen your resolve) and gradually work up from there. Eventually your baby will enjoy tummy time and play in this position.

How can I exercise my baby while he is on his tummy?

There are a lot of ways to play with your baby while he is on his tummy.

1. Place yourself or a toy just out of your baby's reach during playtime to get him to reach for you or the toy.
2. Place toys in a circle around your baby. Reaching to different points in the circle will allow him to develop the appropriate muscles to roll over, scoot on his belly, and crawl.
3. Lie on your back and place your baby on your chest. He will lift his head and use his arms to try to see your face.
4. While being watched by an adult or caregiver, have a young child play with the baby while on his tummy. Young children can get down on the floor easily. They generally have energy for playing with babies, may really enjoy their role as the "big kid," and are likely to have fun themselves.

Bedding

Infants who die from SIDS are more likely to have slept on a pillow or soft mattress and are found with their nose and mouth completely covered by bedding. Soft bedding, in fact, increases the risk of SIDS 5-fold. In addition, babies can suffocate when their faces are next to soft bedding. To eliminate the risk of SIDS and suffocation due to soft bedding, the AAP, US Consumer Product Safety Commission, and National Institute of Child Health and Human Development have revised their recommendations for placing infants to sleep. These organizations recommend that infants younger than 12 months be placed to sleep in a crib with a firm mattress and no soft bedding of any kind. They suggest that parents use one-piece sleepers or other sleep clothing, with no other covering, as an alternative to blankets. If you feel like you need to use a blanket, make sure that it is a thin blanket, tuck it around the crib mattress, reaching only as far as your baby's chest, to reduce the risk of getting his head covered by the bedding.

SLEEPING POSITION AND HEAD SHAPE

Parents and caregivers often worry about their baby developing a flat spot on the back of his head because of sleeping on the back. Though it is possible for a baby to develop a flat spot on his head, it usually rounds out as the baby grows older and sits up. There are ways to reduce the risk of babies developing a flat spot.

1. Alternate which end of the crib you place the baby's feet. This will cause her to naturally turn toward light or objects in different positions, which will lessen the pressure on one particular spot on her head.
2. When baby is awake, vary her position. Limit time spent in freestanding swings, bouncy chairs, and car safety seats. These items all put added pressure on the back of a baby's head.
3. Spend time holding the baby in your arms as well as watching her play on the floor, on her tummy and on her back.
4. A breastfed baby may feed from both breasts during a feeding. You can switch the side where she starts feeding. If the baby is bottle-fed, switch the arm that you use to hold her during feeding.

Your Baby's Room and Crib

Your baby's bedroom and crib or bed should be extra safe. Her crib and—once she's mobile—her room are where she will first push the boundaries of exploration, without direct supervision much of the time. To keep the path clear, her surroundings should be free of traps and hazards as much as possible.

Check that all furniture complies with up-to-date safety requirements and is appropriate for your baby's age. This is especially important when you are using previously owned pieces bought or passed on as gifts. Antique cribs, for example, may look pretty, but the spacing between the slats rarely conforms to the current standard of 2⅜ inches or less, which is intended to make it impossible for a baby's head to become caught. In addition, the finish may include old layers of lead-based paint. You can trust new furniture if it bears the Juvenile Products Manufacturers Association safety certification seal. All fabrics used in your baby's room (for example, sleepwear, sheets, curtains) should be flame retardant.

Selecting a Crib

- Bars should be spaced no more than 2⅜ inches apart.
- The mattress should be very firm and should not sag under your baby's weight. It should fit snugly, with no space between it and the crib walls.
- The top of the crib rail should be at least 26 inches from the top of the mattress. Periodically lower the mattress as your child gets taller.
- The headboards and footboards should be solid, with no decorative cutouts. Corner posts that could cause injury or snag clothing should be removed.
- Do not use cribs with drop rails. These are not safe.
- Crib bumpers (or bumper pads) may seem as though they can help protect babies from drafts and bumps, but they should not be used in cribs. There is no evidence that bumper pads can prevent serious injuries, and they pose a risk of suffocation, strangulation, or entrapment. In addition, older babies can use them for climbing out of the crib.
- Keep large toys and stuffed animals out of the crib, as your baby may use them to get a leg up and over the rail. Pillows, bulky comforters, and heavy blankets do not belong in a crib; a baby can smother under them.

- Place the crib away from windows, where direct sunlight and drafts can make your baby uncomfortable. A crib can become uncomfortably hot if placed too near a radiator. Also make sure that there are no strings from blinds or curtains close by that can wrap around the baby's neck.
- Once your child is about 3 feet tall, he should start sleeping in a bed. If you are worried about him falling out of bed, you may want to start with the mattress on the floor.
- Fit your baby's crib with a firm mattress and make sure there's no space between the mattress and crib walls. Your baby should never sleep on a water bed, sheepskin, pillow, sofa, armchair, or other soft surface. Thick blankets, duvets, comforters, pillows, and large, soft, stuffed toys should never be used in babies' cribs; a baby can easily be smothered if trapped under bulky bedding or when his face is pressed up against a pillow.
- Babies do not need extra support, such as from rolled blankets or commercial devices, to keep them on their backs. Cumbersome materials like these clutter up the crib and may be hazardous for a baby.

HOW LONG SHOULD BABIES SLEEP ON THEIR BACKS?

Now that my 5-month-old baby is rolling over by himself, is it safe to let him sleep on his tummy? If not, what is the best way to keep him on his back?

The American Academy of Pediatrics recommends that parents place healthy babies on their backs to sleep until 1 year of age to reduce the risk of sudden infant death syndrome. However, once a baby can roll over comfortably from back to stomach and stomach to back (this generally happens between 4 and 7 months), there's probably no need to roll him back onto his back if he has rolled over. You should, however, double-check to make sure that there is nothing else in the crib with him. Babies can accidentally roll into pillows, quilts, or bumper pads and suffocate.

Temperature

Babies should be kept warm, but they shouldn't get overheated. Overheating carries an increased risk of SIDS. Make sure the crib isn't positioned next to a radiator, which can quickly heat up the bedding. Also, keep the temperature of the room comfortable and on the cool side. If the baby is sweating or has damp hair, flushed cheeks, or a heat rash, she is getting too hot.

Sleepwear

Babies should be dressed appropriately for the environment. Use no more than one additional layer than an adult would wear to be comfortable. At night, change your baby out of day clothes and into flame-retardant sleepwear. Many parents prefer to dress their babies in an all-in-one sleeper that can be zipped up. This keeps baby comfortably warm and does away with the need for covers, which eliminates the risk of baby becoming tangled and smothering under blankets.

SWEATING IN A SLEEPING BABY

When I go to kiss my baby after she's asleep, I find her damp with sweat. Is this normal?

Some people sweat during the deepest stage of non-rapid eye movement sleep (see Chapter 7, "Rapid Eye Movement Versus Non-Rapid Eye Movement Sleep," on page 110). During these stages, a sleeper has regular, steady breathing and heart rate. Our bodies experience the most restorative effects of sleep at these times. You may find that your baby sweats until her clothes are damp. Usually, this is quite normal and no action is required. However, check to make sure that your baby is not overdressed and that she is not overheated because, for instance, the room is too warm. (This is especially important if your child is younger than 1 year, as overheating is a risk factor for sudden infant death syndrome.) Also check that your baby is not in any distress and that she does not seem to have a high fever. If all is well, simply wipe off your baby's brow and head to prevent her from becoming chilled and let her continue sleeping.

Other Considerations

Breastfeeding

The AAP recommends exclusive breastfeeding for the first 6 months and continued breastfeeding for at least 12 months or as long as baby and mother want to continue. Human milk provides antibodies and other immune-building and protective factors that help safeguard children against infections until their own immune systems are mature enough to take over. Equally important, the AAP recommends breastfeeding as one of the protective factors that can reduce the risk of SIDS. The risk of SIDS is one quarter for a baby who exclusively breastfeeds and half for any baby who breastfeeds.

> **SLEEPING IN CHILD CARE**
>
> The same precaution about placing babies to sleep on their back to minimize the risk of sudden infant death syndrome (SIDS) should be followed in child care settings, where 15% to 20% of all SIDS cases occur—a disproportionately high rate. Be sure that you talk with your child care provider (or anyone else who cares for your baby) to make certain that babies are placed to sleep on their backs and that all other safe sleep recommendations are followed.

Pacifiers

Studies have consistently shown that pacifiers can protect against SIDS, although the mechanism for doing so is not known. Nevertheless, the AAP recommends that parents consider offering their babies a pacifier at nap time and bedtime through the first 6 months and wean off pacifier use by 12 months of age. A pacifier should not be used by a breastfed baby until breastfeeding is firmly established, typically by 3 to 4 weeks of age. If your baby doesn't like the pacifier, don't worry about it. Don't force him to use it. You can try again later.

Sitting Devices

A sitting apparatus should not be used for routine sleep at home or in the hospital before discharge. These devices include car safety seats, strollers, infant carriers, and infant slings. Babies younger than 4 months are particularly at risk because they may end up in positions that make it more difficult to breathe. When you use infant slings and cloth carriers for your baby, make sure that your baby's head is up and above the fabric, her face is visible, and her mouth and nose are not being obstructed. If you are breastfeeding your baby in a sling or cloth carrier, make sure to reposition baby after breastfeeding so that her head is up and above the fabric again.

Bassinets and Cradles

For the first few weeks of a baby's life, some parents prefer to use a bassinet or cradle because it's portable and allows the baby to sleep in their bedroom. But keep in mind that babies grow fast and a cradle that's sturdy enough for a 1-month-old may be outgrown by the next month.

Make sure the bottom of the cradle or bassinet is well supported to prevent its collapse. The cradle or bassinet should also have a wide base so it won't tip over even if someone bumps it; if it has folding legs, make certain that they're locked straight whenever it is being used.

In general, your baby should move to a crib around the end of the first month of life or by the time he weighs 10 pounds.

Bed Sharing

Nursing mothers in many cultures sleep with their babies until they wean. The AAP, however, has expressed concern that bed sharing as it is generally practiced in Western cultures is hazardous. There has been a recent increase in baby deaths, particularly suffocation and strangulation deaths, while bed sharing. Bed sharing is especially dangerous if the bed-sharing parent is using any substances that may alter her ability to wake up, such as pain medications, mind-altering drugs, or alcohol; either parent is a smoker (even if they're not smoking in bed); other people (including siblings) besides parents are also in the bed; a parent is particularly tired; the baby is younger than 3 months; bed sharing occurs on a water bed, sofa, or armchair; or there are blankets and pillows in the bed.

The AAP recommends that parents have their new babies sleep in the same room as them but on a separate sleep surface, such as a bassinet, playpen, or crib. This makes it easy to feed the baby and keep an eye on him when parents are in their own bed. Parents can bring their baby into bed with them for snuggling and feeding, but when parents start to get sleepy, they should move the baby back into the bassinet or crib. Do not feed babies on sofas or armchairs if there is a chance that the parent feeding the baby might fall asleep; that can be dangerous.

Immunizations

Check with your pediatrician to make sure your baby's immunizations are up to date. Research has shown that immunizations lower the risk of SIDS by 50%.

NO-SMOKING ZONE

Create a smoke-free zone around your baby. Babies and young children exposed to tobacco smoke have more colds and upper respiratory infections as well as a higher risk of sudden infant death syndrome (SIDS). The risk of SIDS is higher for babies whose mothers smoked during pregnancy. No one should smoke in your house or car or anywhere around your baby. In fact, this "don't smoke" recommendation should begin during pregnancy, *before* the baby is born. Alcohol and drug use can also increase your baby's risk for SIDS.

CHAPTER 3

Sleep Associations and Strategies: Babies

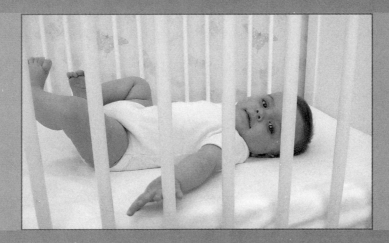

*S*leep is only a step behind feeding among the aspects of baby care most likely to make new parents anxious. Parents are concerned not only about their baby's sleep but also their own. After all, if the baby can't sleep, neither can they.

Most babies sleep for 2 to 3 hours at a time for the first 2 weeks or so, soon extending sleep periods to 4- to 5-hour stretches. This coincides with fewer breastfeeding or bottle-feeding breaks and longer periods of alertness and play. However, well-meaning grandparents and friends may ask, "Is the baby sleeping through the night?" so often that a continuous stretch of nighttime sleep takes on an unrealistic importance. If the magic milestone hasn't appeared by 6 or 8 weeks, the parents wonder if there's something wrong with their baby or the way they are looking after him. Remind your family and friends that a baby who wakes frequently is not a "bad" sleeper. This is a normal part of development. (See Chapter 1 for more information on what it means to be a "good" sleeper.) It is what your baby does on waking that is important. Ideally, when your baby wakes in the middle of the night, he will be able to go back to sleep without needing to call or signal you. "Sleeping through the night" is a misnomer. Everyone, including babies, awakens periodically during the night. Your goal is to help your baby learn how to get himself back to sleep in the middle of the night. Some babies seem to instinctively know how to do this; others need a little coaching from their parents.

In addition, for most babies in the first 6 months of life, sleeping through the night actually means 5 to 6 hours of sleep. So if your 3-month-old goes to sleep at about 8:00 pm, you may expect to be up for the next change and feeding between 1:00 and 3:00 am. Of course, you can adjust this time span by pushing back the last feeding before bedtime. Finally, even after your child has achieved the breakthrough of sleeping through the night, the sleep pattern will change again.

In the early years, most children vary their nighttime routine from time to time. They may sleep undisturbed for weeks or months, then abruptly go back to late-night waking for a while. There are many things that can cause a child to wake up during the night. Teething may be making the baby's mouth sore. The baby may have a viral infection, such as a cold, that throws off his sleep schedule. Or the baby may have taken a leap in development that involves a temporary change in sleeping pattern.

WHY BABIES CRY

Crying is the only way a young baby can make her needs and wants known. It is her way of communicating with you. When your baby cries, she's trying to tell you something or to wind down after a stimulating day; she's not doing it to annoy you. Most parents, in the first few weeks, learn how to tell one kind of cry from another.

Even at this early age, your baby is an individual with certain likes and dislikes (see Chapter 5, "Sleep and Temperament," on page 82), and it's unreasonable to try and control every detail of his behavior. You can't force your child to sleep; what you can do is help him to adjust to daytime and nighttime rhythms that control when he is awake and sleepy. Most importantly, you can help him learn to comfort himself and go back to sleep the several times a night when, like all babies, he awakens but doesn't need to be fed or changed.

Babies and children thrive on a regular routine. This doesn't mean that you have to keep to a rigid schedule. Rather, the more your child can look forward to events rolling out in a predictable sequence, the easier it is to cope with occasional exceptions to the rule, such as when bedtime or a meal is unavoidably delayed. It's never too early to teach a child to sleep well or too late to change a bad habit. Children are adaptable and eager to learn. It's up to parents to take the initiative for change and stick to it, even though the adjustment period may be difficult.

Sleeping Through the Night

If your child is not sleeping 5 to 6 hours through the night by 3 months, there may be a reason. Is her longest sleep time during the daytime or early evening? If so, you may help the process along by keeping her awake longer in the afternoon and early evening. Make sure she has plenty of stimulation during her waking periods—toys, perhaps a "busy box," a brightly patterned rug to lie on, music to listen to, and most of all, someone to talk with. This may help stop her from being lulled into sleep earlier than necessary. Do not expect that you can suddenly change her normal bedtime from 9:00 pm to midnight in one day; you may have to do it gradually over several days.

TOYS IN CRIBS
The safest crib is one with just the baby in it. Pillows, quilts, comforters, sheepskins, bumper pads, and stuffed toys can cause your baby to suffocate. Research has not shown us when it's 100% safe to have these objects in the crib; however, most experts agree that after 12 months of age these objects pose little risk to healthy babies.

Preventing Bedtime Resistance

Even a baby who is a few weeks old may have trouble winding down after a day crowded with activities and people. Keep bedtime calm, with a regular routine, and avoid stimulating play in the evening. Give your attention to your baby during the bedtime routine and concentrate on low-key activities, such as repetitive songs or nursery rhymes and picture books. When the routine is done, place him still awake in his crib. It's not a good idea to prop your baby on your lap and expect him to become drowsy while you watch a movie or television program. The bright, rapidly shifting images and jarring sounds may overstimulate your baby's still-developing nervous system and keep him awake. Furthermore, it is best to avoid screen time until at least 2 years of age and instead read books and tell stories.

From the beginning, it's wise to place your baby in the crib while he is drowsy but still a little bit awake. This helps him link being in the crib with the pleasant feeling of falling asleep. (Psychologists call this forming a *positive sleep association.*) It also helps to orient the baby when he wakes up so that as time goes on, he will lie quietly for a while, enjoying a little time on his own before calling for attention.

When you have completed the going-to-bed ritual, place your baby in his crib still awake. For the first several months of life, *room sharing,* sleeping in close proximity within view without bed sharing, is recommended to prevent sudden infant death syndrome (SIDS). Say your good-nights and dim the lights (a low-wattage table lamp or night-light may also work for some families). If you have a television in your room, you may want to turn it off when it's bedtime for your baby (you can go to another room to watch if you're not quite ready for sleep yourself yet).

WHEN YOUR BABY CRIES AT NIGHT

When your baby cries at night, wait a few minutes to see if she settles down on her own. If not, go to her and try to address her most urgent problem first. For example, if she's cold and hungry and has a wet diaper, put on another layer of clothing to warm her up, change her diaper, then feed her. Keep the lights dim and don't make this into playtime. However, if her crying has a desperate quality, suggesting she's in pain, quickly check on her. One fairly common, but not often looked for, reason for crying is a strand of hair wound around a finger or toe.

When your baby is calm again but still awake, put her back in her crib, say your good-nights, and leave her side. If she cries again after you leave, give her a few minutes to settle on her own. Many babies go to sleep more quickly if left for a while. If the crying keeps up, repeat your visits at increasingly longer intervals, but no longer than 10 minutes at a time. Keep the room dim, speak quietly and no more than you have to, and avoid picking your baby up.

Waking at Night After 4 or 5 Months

Opinions differ about the "right" way to manage nighttime awaking from about the middle of the first year. At one end of the scale is the belief that you should settle the baby and then return to your bed, not going back to the baby except to rescue her in a life-threatening emergency. The baby should be left to cry it out, no matter how long "it" may take. The philosophy here is that the more you leave your baby to cry, the sooner she'll forget that you used to pick her up when she cried. This approach, though, is difficult for most families to fully embrace.

At the other extreme is the school of thought that babies should always fall asleep at the breast or with a bottle, preferably in the parents' bed, and that the baby should be offered a feeding whenever she stirs during the night. This approach is also concerning. For one, bed sharing can be hazardous and is not recommended by the American Academy of Pediatrics (AAP). Babies who sleep in the same bed as their parents are at higher risk of SIDS, suffocation, or strangulation. Parents can roll onto babies during sleep, babies can get tangled in sheets or blankets, or babies can fall and get stuck between the mattress and the wall. While the AAP recommends that new babies sleep in close proximity to their parents, the baby should be on a separate sleep surface, such as a bassinet. (Read about the risks that may be associated with bed sharing in "Sharing a Bed With Your Baby" on page 54.)

In addition, while falling asleep at the breast is a profoundly satisfying experience for a young child, breastfed babies who are allowed to nurse at will during the night may continue to awake for night feedings long after the nutritional need has passed. The breast becomes a pacifier; without it, the baby has difficulty settling down to sleep. This occurs with bottle-fed babies as well. If falling asleep while nursing or drinking from the bottle is the routine, the baby, when she has a normal awakening in the middle of the night, will not be able to fall asleep again without the breast or bottle. It then becomes very difficult to break this routine. Finally, feeding the baby at bedtime or in the middle of the night can promote tooth decay and ear infections.

MAINTAINING A 24-HOUR CYCLE

Natural biological, or circadian, rhythms—including the sleep/wake cycle—follow a 24-hour cycle, but left unregulated, the timing of the rhythms may shift later. Circadian rhythms are helped by a consistent routine with regular cues for activities and functions. Waking at about the same time every morning is an important cue for keeping circadian rhythms keyed to a 24-hour day.

To ensure peaceful nights for everyone, it's probably easier to follow a middle path. It isn't necessary to rush to your baby the moment you hear a whimper, but neither do you and your baby have to suffer increasingly distressed sobs for hours on end. Babies normally cry out or babble during periods of semi-arousal several times every night. In almost all cases, they go back to sleep on their own. As you get to know your baby, you soon learn to distinguish the fussing sounds as she settles down, her hunger cry, the sad cries that tell you she is distressed, and an angry bellow for attention.

If your child needs a clean diaper or other care, provide what she needs with minimum disturbance: Keep the lights dim, speak softly and no more than you need to, change the diaper and place the baby right back in her crib (or change her diaper in the crib if you can), and quickly return to your bed, as at bedtime. If your baby's crying persists longer than 5 to

10 minutes after you leave, return to her without turning on the light, pat her or gently rub her and quietly tell her it's time to sleep, then leave again. Repeat your visits at progressively longer intervals within the 5- to 10-minute range and be firm: no picking up. If you pick her up, your baby will expect a lengthy cuddle and will redouble her crying when you place her down again; sleepiness will be delayed even further. In most cases, this technique will take more than one night. It generally takes 3 to 5 nights for your baby to fall asleep without too much fuss and stay there for 5 or more hours.

Monitor the crying for any change and manage the inevitable false alarms in the same low-key way. When the baby's crib is in your room, you can easily look to make sure that your baby is *really* all right if you hear a cry that sounds like a distress call.

Common Baby Sleep Problems

Pain and Illness

A range of factors can interfere with sleep starting in the earliest months of life. A baby may wake because of fever and pain due to an ear infection or an upset stomach, such as with mild gastroenteritis. Even a minor illness can have a lasting effect on sleep because while it lasts, the parents are especially responsive to the baby's distress. The baby, in turn, enjoys the extra attention and continues to cry for it after the symptoms have cleared up.

Occasionally, night waking may be caused by a problem that needs medical treatment. Poor sleeping, in combination with vomiting, spitting up large amounts of milk, or abdominal pain, may be due to a milk allergy or irritation caused when acidic stomach contents flow back into the esophagus (gastroesophageal reflux). In cases such as this, or after any illness, once the situation has improved, you may need to help your child relearn how to self-soothe himself back to sleep.

TEETHING PAINS

Discomfort from teething, which may begin as early as 3 months, can wake a baby. The gums around the emerging teeth may be swollen and tender. Give her firm objects to chew on—teething rings or hard, unsweetened teething crackers. Frozen teething toys should not be used; extreme cold can injure your baby's mouth and cause more discomfort. Pain relievers intended to be rubbed on a baby's gums aren't very helpful; a teething baby drools so much that the medication is quickly washed away. In addition, pediatricians warn that such medications can numb the back of the throat and interfere with your baby's ability to swallow. If your baby is clearly uncomfortable, talk to your pediatrician about a possible course of action. Your pediatrician may suggest that you give a small dose of acetaminophen (eg, Tylenol) or ibuprofen (eg, Advil, Motrin).

When your baby's teeth are coming through, she may also have a very slight increase in temperature. But if her temperature reaches 100.4°F (38°C) or above, it's not because of teething. If your baby has symptoms such as fever, vomiting, or diarrhea while teething, consult your pediatrician to find out whether she has a medical condition requiring treatment.

If your teething baby is irritable, try to make her comfortable, but keep to your usual bedtime routine. Changing the routine, even for a few nights, may only lead to sleep troubles.

Temperament

In time, most babies naturally fall into regular sleep patterns, thanks to an inborn temperament that allows them to easily adapt (also see Chapter 5, "Sleep and Temperament," on page 82). Those who are more difficult to settle may have less well-established biological rhythms, may be more sensitive to stimuli, or may have intense, excitable personalities and cry harder and louder than other babies, thus finding it harder to calm down. Even at an early age, some babies are less adaptable than others, which makes it difficult for them to accept change. A wide temperamental gap between baby and parents—say, an excitable child with a short attention span and a rigidly methodical parent, or a shy, withdrawn child and a loud, extroverted parent—adds to the difficulty of setting routines. Extra patience, more time, and a change in parenting style may be needed to establish regular sleep habits in these highly sensitive babies. Your baby's pediatrician can advise you and may refer you to a counselor or a support group for parents with similar challenges.

LEARNING NEW SLEEP ASSOCIATIONS

My daughter, now 3 months, had reflux when she was born, so she had to be held upright for 10 to 15 minutes after feedings. She would always fall asleep during this time. Even though she no longer has reflux, she has gotten used to being held and now wakes up several times during the night just to be held. After I have held her for 10 minutes she falls back asleep, but she wakes up every 1 to 2 hours to be held again. How do I break her of this habit?

When you held your baby to prevent her stomach contents from flowing back into her esophagus, she enjoyed the sensation of being cuddled or rocked to sleep, and this is what she became used to. Now your challenge is to help her learn new positive sleep associations (see Chapter 1, "The Importance of Sleep Associations," on page 13). Cuddle and quietly play with your baby during your bedtime routine, then put her in her crib sleepy but still awake. Leave her side and return at increasingly longer intervals to pat your baby gently and reassure her with your voice, but don't pick her up. Manage further waking during the night in a similar way: Go to your baby's crib, leave the lights off (except for a night-light), pat your baby, and speak softly to her, but don't pick her up. Leave her side when she is drowsy but still awake. It may take a few nights for her to learn these new positive sleep associations, but be consistent in what you do.

The results of several studies have shown that babies born after a long or difficult labor tend to wake more at night during their first year than babies with uncomplicated births. However, when researchers looked at the reasons, the babies from difficult deliveries were just as healthy as the others; it appeared that these parents were more likely to pick them up more often, which may have reinforced night waking.

Separation Anxiety

Beginning in the second half of the first year, separation anxiety can cause many nights with disrupted sleep. During this stage (which can last for several months), a baby or toddler may wake several times and cry anxiously for one or both parents, often expressing a strong preference for one. A toddler may try to climb out of her crib, cling desperately, and plead to be allowed to sleep in her parents' bed. She isn't being naughty or manipulative. This is a normal stage in children's emotional development and needs to be managed with a loving and consistent approach. Separation anxiety usually fades away somewhere around the second birthday. Until it does, your child may need reassurance several times night after night.

To deal with separation anxiety as a whole, here are a few steps that you can take.

- No matter how young your baby is, let her know in a matter-of-fact way when you have to leave her. Even if you're only going into another room for a minute, tell her, "I'll be right back." One day she'll surprise you with her own "Right back!" when she's leaving you for a while.
- Play peekaboo and games in the mirror; this helps your baby to understand that mommy and daddy go away and come back.
- Create a diversion to distract your baby's attention when you leave. A babysitter can help with that by sharing a new toy, giving your baby a bath, or showing your baby her reflection in the mirror. Then say goodbye and leave as quickly as possible.
- When you go out in the evening, try to use a familiar babysitter. If you must use a new one, ask her to arrive before the child's bedtime and allow a little time for getting acquainted. Many parents make it a rule to employ a regular babysitter one night a week and plan their social activities accordingly. Children usually find it easy to accept such a separation when it is part of a predictable routine.

How Some Difficult Sleep Associations Form

A few common habits that parents fall into, though with the best of intentions, can disrupt the family's sleep by creating sleep associations that can cause problems later.

- Allowing baby to fall asleep while feeding
- Rocking or holding baby while she falls asleep
- Allowing baby to fall asleep in the parents' bed

These practices can result in sleep associations for your baby that make it difficult for her to fall asleep in the middle of the night. In addition, some of these practices can have negative health consequences. For example, allowing a baby to go to sleep with a bottle of human milk, formula, or juice can cause tooth decay, called *nursing bottle caries,* which badly affects not only baby teeth but permanent teeth as well. This practice can also increase the risk of ear infections, a frequent cause of nights with disrupted and lost sleep. In addition, small babies are in danger of suffocation and SIDS when sharing a bed with larger family members, or if a parent falls asleep on a couch or armchair while holding the baby. In addition, these habits hamper the development of self-reliance in the child, and they stop the child and parents from getting a good night's sleep.

GIVE SLEEP A CHANCE

My daughter, who is 7 months, seems to have a problem with falling asleep by herself or staying in her crib at night. She doesn't have a problem with naps during the day. I have tried various ways except for "letting her cry"; I don't feel comfortable with that strategy. She falls asleep in less than a minute when her head touches our mattress, so she sleeps in our bed at night. Now, after 7 months of sharing, I'm not getting enough sleep, my back hurts, and my husband has moved to the couch.

The answer is not to let her cry but rather to let her fall asleep. Your baby falls asleep without difficulty when you leave her in her crib for daytime naps. However, she can't do so at night because she is always moved to your bed before she's asleep. Thus, she's learned that her parent's bed is where she sleeps at night and has become used to going to sleep on your mattress.

Help your baby learn some new sleep associations. Put her in her crib sleepy but still awake. Leave a night-light on or the door ajar so light shines in from the hallway; she may feel uneasy when her room is totally dark. After saying your good-nights, leave her side and give your baby time to settle. If she continues to cry, return at increasingly longer intervals (between 5 and 10 minutes) to pat or rub her and quietly soothe her with your voice, but don't pick her up.

Be consistent to make the learning process easier on your baby. If you pick her up, she will expect to be carried to your bed. When her rhythm is disturbed in this way she is likely to become wide awake and then have to start falling asleep all over again.

CRYING HELPS BABIES UNWIND

Many babies cry quite hard right after their parents leave the bedroom. In most cases, the crying stops abruptly after a few minutes and the baby settles down to sleep. This is the way the baby winds down emotionally after a day crammed with stimulation. Don't rush back to your baby at the first cry. She probably doesn't need attention. On the contrary, she may need a little time on her own to sort out a jumble of feelings and impressions.

Falling Asleep at the Breast or Bottle

"My baby can't settle down to sleep unless she is nursing"; "I have to give my child a bottle or he cries himself to sleep." As noted earlier, these babies have been taught to associate feeding or nursing for comfort and sleeping in such a way that the breast or bottle and the mother are part of the going-to-sleep routine and the baby cannot fall asleep without them. Some pediatricians describe the mothers of such babies as "too good" because they do so much more than the child wants or needs. By anticipating every whim, they may prevent their children from developing a natural ability to soothe themselves.

For some infants and their mothers, a final feeding is a comforting, calming part of the preparing-for-bed routine. Breastfeeding may be nonnutritive and your baby may be used to finding comfort in breastfeeding as a pacifier. While this is a normal way for babies to find comfort, routinely breastfeeding as the last activity of night will often create an undesired habit. For bottle-feeding babies, the bottle should not be used as a pacifier because it may lead to overfeeding and at bedtime will lead to an unwanted habit. If your baby needs extra comfort from sucking to fall asleep, help him find his thumb or give him a pacifier. Many children suck their thumbs and fingers for comfort while falling asleep and at no other time. More than half of all thumb-suckers stop before the end of their first year. No matter what well-intentioned family members may say, thumb-sucking or pacifier use is a normal habit. Many children eventually wean themselves of the thumb-sucking or pacifier habit without any intervention.

To break the habit of nighttime feeds, most pediatricians recommend phased withdrawal rather than the cold turkey method. When the child wakes during the night, wait a few minutes to see if she will fall back asleep by herself. If the child is older than about 6 months, the amount of milk given at night should be tapered off, the duration of the feeding shortened, and the feedings finally discontinued altogether. For formula-feeding infants older than 6 months, some pediatricians advise diluting nighttime bottle-feedings with water. Start by replacing a quarter of the usual amount of milk or formula with water, and increase the dilution over several nights until the bottle contains nothing but water. At this point, babies generally lose interest and stop waking for the nighttime feeding. A baby may cry less if withdrawal visits are managed by the parent who does not usually provide nighttime feedings and thus is not associated with the routine.

In most cases, it should be possible to complete the withdrawal process within 2 weeks. Once the feedings are stopped, nighttime crying should be managed similarly. Wait a few minutes to see if the baby will fall asleep on his own. If crying continues, visits should be brief and occur at increasingly longer intervals, between 5 and 10 minutes at a time. Speak in a soft, reassuring tone to your baby, pat him or rub him gently, but *don't pick him up.* The sooner you make the change, the easier it will be. However, make sure you choose a time to change the response when your baby doesn't need extra attention because of an illness with uncomfortable symptoms. If you are concerned about letting your baby cry for a longer period than usual because it may wake your other children or disturb the neighbors, choose a weekend or school vacation time when the crying will be less disruptive. If you live in an apartment building, let your neighbors know what you're trying to do so they are aware.

There are parents who simply cannot bear to hear their baby cry, even for a minute or two. In such cases, a workable solution may be to agree on a plan whereby the more sensitive parent uses earplugs, takes a walk, or otherwise keeps busy and leaves the other partner to deal with the bedtime routine.

Rocking a Fussy Baby to Sleep

Few sounds are more upsetting or puzzling to parents than the fussy or colicky crying that comes on without warning in the first few weeks of their baby's life. Colic is marked by hours of inconsolable crying that starts at about the same time every day, lasts for hours, and may be recurrent over weeks. Bouts of colic usually begin when babies are between 2 and 4 weeks old and frequently taper off between 2½ and 4 months, although some babies are still colicky at 6 months. About 1 baby in every 5 develops colic.

Even though not all babies have colic, most have at least a daily period of fussy crying that leaves parents or caregivers feeling helpless and frustrated. While the crying is going on, nothing seems to help, and yet the crying usually stops as abruptly as it started and the baby quickly falls asleep.

The causes of colic and fussy crying are unknown and there is no cure, but all babies eventually outgrow this phase. It may simply be a stage in the maturation of the nervous system during which babies have difficulty processing the vast amount of sensory input they receive each day. Whatever the cause, parents find by trial and error that many colicky babies can be calmed, at least some of the time, by swaddling (wrapping the baby firmly in a receiving blanket), sucking (a breast, bottle, finger, or pacifier), and rhythmic movement (gentle rocking, walking, swinging). Music, white noise—a steady sound supplied by a recording or a radio tuned to static—and the rhythmic sounds of household appliances have all been used successfully to quiet colicky babies. However, what works today for your baby may not work tomorrow, and many parents develop a whole repertory of calming strategies until one day, the colic or fussy crying simply stops.

However, remember that rocking is helpful as long as it is used to calm the baby before she is placed, still awake, in the crib. If babies are regularly rocked to sleep, they come to depend on rocking long after the reason for it—fussy crying or colic—has come and gone. At first you rock because your baby is fussy; later, your baby gets fussy unless you rock. As with offering the breast or bottle, picking up the baby and rocking her every time she whimpers stifles her ability to learn self-soothing skills. Also, keeping your baby aroused with unnecessary attention and movement robs her and you of much-needed rest.

It's understandable that many parents get into a habit of "preventive rocking"; anything to stop the desperate cries of a fussy, colicky baby. But while it's only natural to try to comfort your baby, there's little you can do to prevent or stop the crying bouts. This is a phase that the baby outgrows. Sleep experts agree that factors that disturb sleep in the first several weeks of

---

PARENTS MAY BE OVER-INVOLVED

Sleep problems may start because parents provide unnecessary nighttime feeding, soothing, or other stimulation. As long as these continue, their children will also persist in demanding nonstop entertainment. When parents recognize their contribution to the problem and withdraw the attention, most children accept the change after a short transition period. Children are fast learners who quickly adapt to changes in their routine. They also deserve time on their own without parental intervention to learn how to soothe and occupy themselves.

life, such as colic, are inherent and self-limited, whereas after 4 months, poor sleep habits are learned and not inborn.

Sharing a Bed With Your Baby

The AAP and the US Consumer Product Safety Commission have cautioned that bed sharing is hazardous for children younger than 1 year. Tiny babies can be smothered under bedclothes or the weight of a much larger body (also see Chapter 2, "Bed Sharing," on page 37), they can fall between the mattress and the wall, and they are also at higher risk for SIDS. However, many parents bed share with their babies because it makes it easier to feed the baby in the middle of the night. In addition, bed sharing is a widespread practice in many cultures, and most children suffer no long-lasting ill effects. However, what's often overlooked is that in countries where bed sharing is routinely practiced, families almost never sleep in beds with soft mattresses, pillows, and bulky covers. A baby may be less likely to smother when the family sleeps on a floor mat with only a light coverlet.

Studies in countries where most adults need regular sleep hours to maintain fixed work schedules have shown that parents and children alike have higher quality sleep when they are sleeping in their own beds. Other studies have shown that children who do not get enough sleep over a prolonged period become irritable or emotional and find it hard to concentrate. These effects can show up in lower test scores by the time children reach school age.

Many advocates of cue-based breastfeeding suggest that all babies should sleep with their mothers and nurse at will during the night. Some parents prefer this arrangement, while others find that with an extra body in the bed, it's hard to get enough rest. A "side car" arrangement—the crib placed next to the parents' bed—may be more comfortable and will be safer than bed sharing.

For most families, a crib in the parents' room allows plenty of togetherness with fewer interruptions to sleep. In any case, a nourished baby does not need night feedings after about the first 4 months. Bed sharing may hamper the baby's attempts to develop his own resources, such as thumb-sucking, for getting to sleep.

Safety risks aside, there are many reasons given for bed sharing, and it may be helpful to discuss these with your pediatrician. If the reasons are economic—the parents can't afford a crib for the baby—there may be local programs that can help them purchase a crib or receive one free of charge. If a parent sleeps with the baby to offset loneliness, counseling may be helpful. Occasionally, a baby who bed shares becomes the buffer between partners in a troubled marriage. Again, counseling could help to identify and resolve the problem.

Time to Sleep

A consistent approach to bedtime may not prevent your baby from waking at night, but it can keep temporary changes in the baby's pattern from developing into a full-scale sleep disorder. We've mentioned some of these suggestions already, but from the start, place your baby to sleep in a room that is dark, quiet, and a comfortable temperature. Avoid rough play and stimulating activities in the hour before bedtime. Develop a bedtime routine that emphasizes calm, soothing activities, such as stories and music in the baby's room, and always bring it to a close by placing your baby still awake in the crib and promptly leaving her side. Ignore cries of protest and give your baby time to settle down. When you hear a whimper in the night, give your baby a chance to go back to sleep on her own before checking on her. When you check on her, do it quietly, keeping the light dim and talking no more than necessary. And remember that children are happy and function best when they can look forward to regular schedules for all their needs, including meals, naps, bedtimes, and starting the day's activities.

PLUSES AND MINUSES OF DIFFERENT METHODS FOR GETTING BABIES TO SLEEP		
Method	**Pluses**	**Minuses**
Sleep associations (baby put in crib sleepy but awake; parent checks and pats as needed at intervals from 5 to 10 minutes without picking baby up)	• Baby associates crib with pleasant feeling of falling asleep. • Easy to use in any family situation. • Often establishes good sleep habits early on. • Parents feel comfortable knowing their baby is not seriously distressed.	• Baby may find it hard to settle in different surroundings. • May be stressful for some parents. • Scheduled visits may get baby's hopes up and provoke further crying. • Scheduled intervals longer than 10 minutes may result in distress.
Cry it out (no going back except in emergency)	• Baby will fall asleep eventually.	• With prolonged crying, baby may become too upset to sleep. • Can be stressful to hear baby crying for long periods. • Noise level may be intolerable.
Bed sharing (baby sleeps on same surface as another person)	• Can facilitate night feedings. • Enhances parent-infant bonding.	• Danger of suffocation. • Hazardous for young babies because of soft sleep surfaces, loose bedding, and increased risk of SIDS/suffocation. • May unnecessarily prolong night feedings. • Neither parent nor baby gets adequate steep. • May make it difficult for baby to adapt to his own bed. • May mask parental problems that need attention.

Abbreviation: SIDS, sudden infant death syndrome.

CHAPTER 4

Toddlers

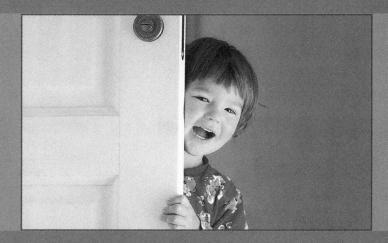

*A*s infants become toddlers, they change physically, emotionally, and socially. They are busy exploring the world and will often need help in "winding down" before sleep.

Once you move through your baby's first year, perhaps with some sleep deprivation of your own along the way, you have almost certainly noticed some sleep-related characteristics of your baby that will extend into the toddler years. During the second year of life, your child will often be reluctant to go to sleep at bedtime and will put it off for as long as possible. He may argue and delay and try to climb out of his crib, no matter how tired he is. You may have thought that the first time he slept through the night finally put an end to the challenges of bedtime, but you've quickly discovered that this is far from the case.

At times, it may be tempting to just let your child fall asleep in his tracks when exhaustion finally sets in. But that can only make sleep problems worse. You need a consistent, steady approach for the long term.

How Much Sleep Does My Toddler Need?

Toddlers sleep about 10 to 13 hours out of the 24 in a day. The exact duration of your toddler's nighttime sleep may vary with her temperament, activity level, health, and growth. But children at the toddler stage are curious and social by nature. Once they can climb out of their cribs or beds, they may also seem to be convinced that there's a party going on somewhere in the house and want to join in the fun.

Many parents go through a difficult phase of trying to keep their toddler in bed, especially around the time she switches to a regular bed. The best way to deal with this phase is to respond calmly to reasonable requests (such as for a drink of water), let your toddler see that nothing special is going on, and return her gently but firmly to bed each time she pops out.

Most toddlers still have an afternoon nap. They take naps of 2 to 3 hours in length about midday, although some may take 2 shorter naps instead. But even when a child does not sleep, it's still a good idea to have a quiet period, perhaps with time to read a story in the early afternoon. This pattern may continue well into the preschool years; preschools and kindergartens usually have a rest period sometime during the school day.

TODDLERS: FORMING GOOD SLEEP HABITS

For parents of toddlers, bedtime is frequently the most challenging part of the day. Toddlers often resist going to sleep, particularly if older siblings in the household are still awake. Here are some tips to help your toddler establish good sleep habits.

1. *Adopt a nightly routine* so your child has quiet time before bedtime and understands that it will soon be time to go to sleep. The routine should be the same each night, as toddlers are comforted by routine. Give her a bath, read her a story, or listen to soft music. Avoid active play, which will only excite her and make sleep more difficult.
2. *Be consistent.* Bedtime should be at the same time every night. By doing so, your child will know what to expect, and it will help her establish good sleep habits.
3. *Let your toddler take a favorite object to bed at night*—perhaps a teddy bear, special blanket, or favorite toy. It can help her fall asleep—and fall back asleep if she awakens during the night. Make sure the object has no buttons or ribbons that could put your child at risk for choking.
4. *Make certain your toddler is comfortable.* If she wants a drink of water or a night-light turned on, do so and then tell her it's time for sleep.
5. *Do not let your child sleep in your bed.* Doing so makes it more difficult for her to fall asleep when she's alone.
6. *Wait several seconds* before you go into your toddler's room whenever she complains or calls out. Then each time she calls for you, wait a little bit longer before you respond. Reassure your child that you are there, even when you're out of sight. Each time you respond, remind her that it's time for her to go to sleep. Don't do anything to reward your child for calling out for you.
7. *Give it time.* It's normal to become upset if your child keeps you awake at night. But try to be understanding, or you're likely to make the problem with sleep even worse. You may need to ask for help from your partner and other adults again when your toddler has sleep disruptions.

So what can you do to promote sound sleep in your toddler? The first step is to create a sleep schedule for your child. When you see that she's tired, make that her bedtime. Then build a sleep routine around this time. You can have her take a bath, read a story, or sing a song, followed by some quiet time before you leave the room so she can sleep.

But even once routines are in place, you can't always rely on your toddler to sleep through a nap period or the nighttime. In addition to being unpredictable in childhood, sleep can also be disrupted by events like changing rooms or beds, losing a favorite blanket or cuddly toy, or going on a family vacation. Keeping to a regular bedtime routine makes it easier to cope with occasional exceptions to the schedule. When bedtime is delayed, settle your child with a shorter version of the usual going-to-bed routine.

CHANGING A TRANSITIONAL OBJECT

My 16-month-old uses my hair as a comfort object and continually runs his hands through it to fall asleep when he wakes in the middle of the night. How can I get him to learn to comfort himself on his own?

Because your toddler is used to the texture and odor of your hair, he may more easily accept a transitional object that simulates one or both of those features. Try giving him a small furry teddy bear or another cuddly toy, and dress it in one of your old T-shirts. When he awakens in the night, check that he is comfortable and then go back to your own bed. The more you pick him up and linger, the more you encourage him to play with your hair.

Challenges in Sleeping Through the Night

There are a number of issues to keep in mind as you help your toddler sleep better. One of them is *independence versus clinginess.* There is a surge of independence that accompanies your child's mastery of walking. But it may be overtaken by a return to clinginess around 18 months of age. Psychologists have suggested that this stage may be a reaction to the toddler's growing awareness of separation. Attachment to transitional objects is more intense now than at any other stage. The teddy bear, blanket, or whatever the favorite item may be is a stand-in for the parent or caregiver and helps the child make the crossover to symbolic thinking.

At around 2 years, the toddler's mixed feelings about his increasing independence can lead to more oppositional behavior, where his resounding "No!" is the usual response, sometimes accompanied by vigorous head nodding, indicating his real wish to say "Yes." Crying and emotional outbursts may be everyday events for a while at bedtime and other times of the day. When your toddler flings himself on the floor, kicking and fighting, remind yourself that this is part of normal development. It does not reflect badly on him or your ability as a parent. Toddlers have tantrums to communicate an unmet emotional need.

Try to keep your toddler's tantrums within limits. Make sure that he doesn't become over-tired, overstimulated, or unnecessarily frustrated by developmentally inappropriate expecta-tions or situations. Set reasonable guidelines for behavior. Children are more likely to have tantrums if parents are too strict or fail to set any limits at all. Children are also more likely to have tantrums when they are overtired, hungry, or thirsty. This frustrating phase may stretch from 1 to 4 years of age.

When bedtime is difficult at this age—with resistance, repeated curtain calls, and occasional tantrums—how should you respond? Do so in a matter-of-fact way. Stay calm and reassur-ing, then leave the room. Or if your toddler seems fearful and becomes unusually upset when you leave, sit quietly with him for a while, then try the "vanishing chair routine" (see box below). On successive nights, gradually move your chair closer toward the doorway, until it's finally outside the room.

VANISHING CHAIR ROUTINE

One method to help foster sleep independence in your child is with the vanishing chair routine. Begin by sitting in your child's room several nights in a row. Each night, move your chair a little farther away from your child's bed until you are sitting outside the room, in the hallway, still within your child's earshot and prepared to respond to her cries. Finally, when she is used to seeing you go out of the room to get to the chair, you will no longer have to keep sitting in the chair to reas-sure her.

Remember, toddlers are also creatures of habit. They thrive on routines—not only going-to-bed routines but also regular schedules for meals and snacks, going for walks, story time, and the 101 activities that fill their days. If a routine is disrupted—short-term or temporary disruptions like a change in bedroom during a home renovation or a trip or vacation away from home, or more lasting issues like losing or misplacing a nighttime cuddly toy—even a normally easygoing toddler may become upset. So keep to your regular routines without being rigid about it. It's equally important to help your child learn to adhere to routines and learn to deal with change when necessary.

TODDLER WAKES EVERY NIGHT

Why does my 16-month-old wake at the same time every night?

Your toddler seems to be waking out of habit. Perhaps he was used to feeding at the same time every night. Or is he disturbed by a sound or light cue that occurs regularly?

Waking at night isn't rare among children—it occurs in as many as 30% of 2-year-olds. It becomes a problem when the child does not or cannot go back to sleep on his own. It sometimes happens in children who have so-called "circadian rhythm problems" that may be a sign of a chaotic home life and unpredictable routines in which children set their own schedules, including when and how long they sleep.

The human body operates on an internal clock functioning on cycles of about 24 hours (known as circadian rhythms), but these cycles can be disrupted by outside influences—from exposure to light to food and exercise. When a child who is out of rhythm finally does get to sleep, he may be hard to wake up in the morning and does not behave as though he is well rested.

Your toddler may also be waking up because of a sleep association. Perhaps he is used to falling asleep while you are holding him or while he is watching television.

So how should you respond to a child with sleep disruptions like this? If the cause of his waking and difficulty sleeping is unwanted sound or light, make any necessary environmental changes. These could include adding white noise, modifying the activities of family members (for example, keeping the television quieter, running the bath at a different time), installing shades to block out light, or asking family members to keep their voices low in an adjoining room. Review his typical bedtime routine to see if there is a sleep association that is the problem.

You may need to give him new sleep associations. You should have a consistent routine leading up to bedtime, then place him in the crib while he is still awake (ideally, he will be a little drowsy) so that he will learn to fall asleep on his own. You could also try giving him a soft toy or blanket to hold as he is falling asleep. He may cry initially, which will necessitate you going in to check on him and reassure him every 10 minutes or so. But if you are consistent, within a few nights he should be falling asleep without too much of a fuss—and be able to get himself back to sleep after he awakes in the middle of the night.

What Else Can Disrupt Sleep?

In toddlers, teething sometimes interferes with sleep, as do colds or upper respiratory infections, which are especially common at this age. Other conditions such as apnea or allergies might be an issue. For more information on these and other health concerns, see Part 2: Childhood Sleep Challenges beginning on page 139.

COUGH AND COLDS: WHAT *NOT* TO DO
Over-the-counter cough and cold medicines should not be given to babies, infants, and children younger than 2 years because of the risk of life-threatening side effects. Also, several studies show that cold and cough products don't work in children younger than 6 years and can have potentially serious side effects. We would recommend not giving any of these medications to your child unless you have been instructed to do so by your pediatrician.

Nightmares also can begin during the toddler years and are especially common during periods of stress, such as toilet training or the arrival of a new baby. Many toddlers begin to recount vivid dreams almost as soon as they can string a simple sentence together, and nightmares are particularly scary to a young child who may not yet be able to draw the line between the real world and her imagination. Comfort your toddler, reassure her that she is safe and protected from "dangers" that may have surfaced in her dreams, and return her to her bed when she's calm but still awake.

During the daytime, try to minimize sources of stress. Bad dreams are not usually a sign of trouble, but if they occur frequently enough to make you concerned or your child's sleep is often broken up by nightmares, talk it over with your pediatrician. (Also see Chapter 11, Nightmares, Night Terrors, and Other Partial Arousals.)

Illness and Recuperation

Babies and young children may have problems sleeping when they are sick. Their rest period is broken by discomfort caused by fever, pain, coughing, runny or stuffy nose, and other symptoms. A stuffed-up nose can be particularly irksome because young babies do not like to breathe through their mouths. Even when a baby breathes through his mouth, he may have trouble feeding and can't soothe himself by sucking his thumb. A sick child usually has trouble falling asleep and staying asleep. This is especially frustrating because a long, restful sleep often seems to help a child turn the corner from feeling ill to getting better. It is no different than when you have a cold.

For as long as symptoms are present, your sick child will need soothing, cuddling, possibly frequent cleanups, drinks, medication, and whatever comfort you can provide to help him sleep. Of course, call your pediatrician if your baby younger than 3 months (12 weeks) has a fever, with temperature of 100.4°F (38°C) or higher, or if your child has severe or persistent symptoms at any age.

As soon as your child is well again, pick up your normal nighttime routine. Lights go out at the regular time and everybody stays quietly in bed unless there's a real problem needing attention. If you're attentive when your child needs you and consistent but not inflexible about limits, he will go along with the system. A young baby may continue to wake up periodically during the night because he has quickly become used to the extra attention and cuddling he enjoyed while sick. However, your calm and consistent approach will help him get back to the usual routine. Once he has had a few bouts with common childhood illnesses—colds, ear infection, or gastroenteritis—he will understand that rules can be bent when a person doesn't feel well. He'll be glad to get back to the normal routine as he feels better.

Body Rocking and Head Banging

Rhythmic, repetitive activity at bedtime is a common early childhood behavior that seems to calm the child even as it mystifies parents. It's hard to understand how a toddler could derive comfort from rocking back and forth on all fours while knocking his head into the railings of his crib, sitting up and bumping his upper body against the headboard, or lying face down and banging his head on the mattress. Nevertheless, a small percentage of young children soothe themselves in this way for about 15 minutes and even longer while preparing for sleep. Children usually outgrow rocking, rolling, and head banging between 18 months and 3 years of age. It can be distressing for parents but is generally harmless. While it may occasionally result in a minor bump, bruise, or callus, severe injury is rare. If the activity continues, becomes more intense, or occurs in the daytime, ask your pediatrician for an evaluation.

> **MASTURBATION IN A YOUNG CHILD**
>
> **We adopted our 5-year-old son at age 3½. He frequently masturbates while in bed. One book we consulted described this as** *infantile pseudo-masturbation.* **Is it simply a comforting habit—like thumb-sucking—that will recede as he develops, or could it indicate a more serious psychological problem?**
>
> Masturbation, or stimulation of the genitals, is normal and common among boys and girls. For most young children, masturbation is just a comforting sensation. Parents should neither discourage nor call unnecessary attention to the activity. However, if your son stimulates himself in public, talk with him about the inappropriateness of this behavior in public.
>
> At times, excessive masturbation or a public display may be a sign that a child is under emotional strain, has poor impulse control, is unduly preoccupied with sex, or is not receiving the emotional comfort he needs. In some cases it may indicate that a child has been sexually abused. Make sure that your child does not have access to sexual material and is not exposed to inappropriate nudity in your home.
>
> If there is a compulsive quality to your child's activity; if he has signs of emotional disturbance, such as fecal soiling, aggressiveness, or social withdrawal; or if you have any concerns about the influence of other children or adults with whom your child has been spending time, consult your pediatrician, who will examine your child and recommend an appropriate course of action.

More Thoughts on Sleep Solutions

From birth to age 5 years, the one thing parents can count on is change. Young children switch back and forth, sleeping through the night for weeks or months at a time, then passing through phases of troubled, fitful nights when the whole family feels cranky because of sleep loss. In the wakeful times, you may feel desperate enough to try a number of tactics that you may have heard about, such as driving around the neighborhood in the early morning hours or running your vacuum cleaner, hoping that your still-alert toddler will fall asleep.

As a general rule, however, your child will settle down with the measures that are woven into your bedtime routine. Like most parents, you will develop a system by trial and error. It may incorporate bits and pieces of several methods, along with advice from your pediatrician and scraps of family lore. Above all, trust your instincts. You know by now what makes your child comfortable. What counts in the end is whether you and your child get a good night's sleep and wake up refreshed and ready for work and play.

Regardless of any advice you may be offered, you will discover approaches that work not only for your family but for each child within your family. What works for one may not help another; much depends on factors like the child's temperament, birth order, and family dynamics.

One technique does not work for all children all the time, with no exceptions. Such rigidity applied to sleeping, eating, and other natural functions can evolve into tools for controlling children, rather than encouraging them to develop as individuals with their own internal systems of behavioral checks and balances.

HUNGER WAKES A TODDLER

At 20 months of age, my son is still waking up at 2- to 3-hour intervals every night. He usually asks for a drink of juice or something to eat. His daytime care provider has trouble getting him to eat because he drinks a lot of juice and then has no appetite for food.

Your son may well be waking up because he's hungry. Some toddlers drink so much that they have no appetite for food. Juices fill your child up but don't provide the nourishment of solid foods. Limit juice to no more than 4 ounces a day and offer it only with a meal or snack. His appetite may improve if you offer water instead of juice when he's thirsty. You can stop buying juice and let him know that he can have water instead. Or you can cut down gradually over a week or two by giving slightly smaller servings each time he asks for juice and diluting it with increasing amounts of water. Give your child's care provider clear instructions about the feeding schedule and between-meal drinks.

TIPS FOR A RESISTANT SLEEPER

In her blog, *Confessions of a Dr. Mom,* pediatrician Melissa Arca, MD, FAAP, offers tips that have worked for her family and may work for you depending on the age and temperament of your child.

Keep an open door

When our son was 4 and still calling us into his room at 3:00 am, we finally came up with this solution: we laid out some blankets and a pillow on the floor next to our bed in our room. We told him that if he woke up and could not get back to sleep, he was welcome to come in and sleep there, but to please *not* wake us up.

It worked. Some mornings I'd find him sleeping right there on the floor or he'd still be sleeping snug in his own bed. Simply having that option put his mind at ease and he was more likely to sleep through the night.

Pillow talk

Be honest with your child. Discuss the importance of sleep and put it in terms they can grasp. They need sleep to grow taller, get smarter, and kick that ball really far. Without it, their bodies and brains don't feel as good. Not to mention the effect it has on Mommy and Daddy…happy well-rested parents are more apt to read that extra bedtime book or stay an extra 20 minutes at the park.

Worry jar

My son had soooo many questions and concerns…of course right at bedtime. This would inevitably prolong the time to lights out and increase the number of times he got out of bed. We started having him write down his "worries" on pieces of paper and putting them in his own worry jar. His worries were put to bed…so we could finally put him to bed too.

Bunk up

In another attempt to survive the bedtime routine without succumbing to sleep ourselves, we decided to move Little Sister into Big Brother's room. That way, they would both have company and not be alone. There was a bit of transition with Big Brother keeping Little Sister awake (when she's tired, she's tired…no resistance here). But soon, they both grew to love the nighttime company and our resistant little sleeper slept a little better.

Managing a Midnight Rambler

Toddlers who have just graduated from a crib to a bed are often intoxicated by the sense of freedom this new status brings. They get into bed willingly enough, then get out again before they've given themselves a chance to become drowsy and start falling asleep. A toddler can easily make 20 or more "farewell appearances" in an evening.

Several questions arise with this new stage of mobility. First, will your child continue to sleep in a crib? Or is it time to switch to a bed? And whether she remains with her crib a while longer or graduates to a bed, how do you persuade her to stay there the whole night through?

You may be able to keep a toddler in a crib for a few months longer by lowering the crib mattress as far as it will go, so that the rail is too high to climb over. (Raised crib sides should be at least 26 inches above the mattress support in its lowest position.) It's also essential to remove crib bumpers and bulky stuffed toys, which children use to get a leg up; in fact, these items should never be placed in the crib in the first place (for tips on crib safety, see "Selecting a Crib" on page 33). Some parents resort to crib tents, available commercially, which form a ceiling over the top of the crib. However, these products may pose a suffocation or head entrapment risk. Some children may also feel uncomfortably confined when their movements are restricted in this way.

IF AT FIRST YOU DON'T SUCCEED…

We have a 3-year-old son and not one night goes by without his waking up and coming into our room to sleep. I'll bring him back to his room 3 or 4 times before I finally give up and lose the battle. Is there any way we can all get a good night's sleep?

Your question suggests that you already know the answer. As you say, you "finally give up and lose the battle," and in doing so you teach your 3-year-old that persistence is the key to success. He knows that after 3 or 4 trial runs, he will eventually get what he wants. To reprogram the behavior, you will have to demonstrate similar persistence and return your son to his bed every time he gets out. This may mean a higher level of sleep disturbance for several nights, but your child will catch on. If you prefer to head him off before he reaches your bedroom, try hanging a small bell on his door to wake you when he leaves his room. And if he is unusually persistent, you may have to stay awake long enough to train him with the "vanishing chair routine" (see page 62).

Managing the Switch to a Bed

On transferring permanently to a bed, your toddler may have a heady sense of freedom the first few nights. Luckily, most children are happy to "graduate" and stay in their beds more willingly than they did in their cribs. However, for a few, the transition has to be managed closely (also see "Tips for a Resistant Sleeper" on pages 68–69). The best way is to continue with the same bedtime routine you have used since your child first joined the family (see Chapter 5) and repeat the following steps:

1. When you end a routine, tell your child to stay in bed until you come for her.

2. If she gets out of bed, calmly and quietly lead her back and tell her she must stay in bed.

3. When she gets back into bed, reward her by telling her briefly what a good girl she is for being there, then leave the room.

4. Tell her that you will come and check on her during the night. For some children it provides reassurance.

THAT'S THE TICKET!

Rewards, given the morning after a successful all-night stay in bed, are a good way to encourage children to stay in bed. Another useful reward technique is to use tickets. Give your child a certain number of tickets before bed that can be used for "curtain calls." Any unused tickets can be turned in for a reward in the morning.

But don't kid yourself that the struggle is over. Be prepared to repeat steps 1 and 2 as many times as you have to for several nights in a row. Twenty "farewell appearances" in one evening is by no means an unusual number. Above all, stay calm and keep interactions with your child on a low-key level; they should be brief and boring. The aim is to reward her with praise for staying in bed and not for getting out. Children tend to feel, as many advertisers do, that any attention is better than none. If getting out of bed brings your toddler extra attention—even negative attention, by making you angry—she'll do it again and again. By contrast, if you keep the atmosphere quiet and even boring, the excitement of getting out will soon pale.

While respecting your toddler's newfound mobility, insist on the rule that once it's time for sleep, people have to stay in bed until morning unless they have to go to the bathroom. Avoid rewarding bedroom breakouts, such as by allowing your child to climb into your bed or join the members of the family who are still up. Instead, praise her in the morning for having stayed in bed all night.

Making Climbers Safer

If your child is going to climb out of bed whether you want him to or not, let him know that the only time that climbing out is acceptable is when sleep or nap time is over. In addition, you should make his room as safe and hazard-free as you can. While you are waiting to buy a new bed, place the crib mattress on the floor. Clear away furniture and large toys, like rocking horses, that could injure your child if he fell against them. You may need to install a safety gate across your toddler's bedroom door to keep him from wandering when you are not awake. You will also need a gate at the top of the stairs to prevent possible injury when your toddler gets out of bed. Install childproof latches on chests of drawers or tape drawers shut so they can't be pulled out and used as steps.

CHAPTER 5

Bedtime Routines and Rituals

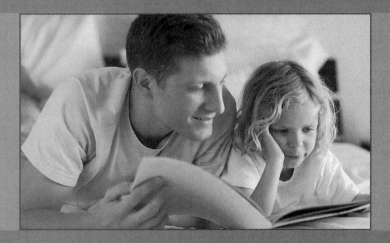

*I*t's almost impossible to overstress the importance of a calm, orderly bedtime routine, but we don't want to suggest that parents should set a fixed routine and stick to it no matter what. Let's talk about multiple bedtime routines rather than a single one.

Four-year-old Katie's mother never varied the schedule: dinner at 6:00 pm, bath at 6:30, play for 15 minutes, then lights out by 7:15, sleepy or not. She was becoming increasingly impatient with Katie's repeated requests for drinks of water, having the door a little more open or a little more closed, and questions about this and that.

Across town, Dylan, a preschool playmate of Katie's, went to sleep and stayed asleep where he dropped off, generally in front of the television. His mother had long since given up nightly struggles to get Dylan to settle into bed and preferred to save her energy for the inevitable morning rush. She kept the peace by simply covering him with a comforter where he lay.

Katie's mother was needlessly strict about scheduling; Katie wasn't ready to sleep at 7:15 pm. If Katie was allowed another 30 minutes or so for reading and quiet play, she would more easily settle for sleep and make fewer "curtain calls."

By contrast, Dylan's mother had never really tried to get Dylan into a regular going-to-bed routine and instead let the television do the job for her. It's not too late to change a poor habit and help Dylan to get ready for bed with quiet time in his bedroom. By keeping evenings more orderly, the family could avoid the troublesome morning rush.

Start With a Routine

Your going-to-bed procedure may vary slightly from day to day, depending on how tired and ready for bed your child seems; however, the basic elements should always be the same. Sometimes, you may skip the bedtime routine altogether, except for cleanup, change, and good-night kiss, when your child is exhausted after a long and action-packed day. Mostly, however, you'll find time to wind down with activities that may include a warm bath, a quiet cuddle, music, stories, and prayers. Avoid scary stories and games involving monster chases or other activities that may be overstimulating. Turn off the television, any video games, and the computer in the hour or so before bedtime and keep interactions calm and soothing.

After Babyhood

As children grow out of babyhood, they can start their bedtime routine by helping with a quick cleanup to put toys and books back in their places and leave the room tidy for the morning. Bedtime also brings lots of opportunities for thoughtful one-on-one talks. However, it is not the time to raise issues that may make your child anxious, such as reproaches for bad behavior or a poor school report.

Even though certain parts of the routine, such as stories or games, may vary from one night to another, it's essential that the "indispensable" steps always be included. Brush your child's teeth or help her to brush them. (Most children need close supervision and help with brushing and flossing until they are about 8 years old—and for a long time afterward, parents may have to remind children to brush their teeth every night and morning until it becomes second nature.) Remind her to use the bathroom one last time if she is toilet trained or even if

---

"ODD JOBS" TO FOSTER INDEPENDENT SLEEPING

My 3-year-old daughter won't go to sleep unless my husband or I stay in the room. She says she's afraid now but will sleep alone when she gets bigger. When do children grow out of this fearful phase?

Your daughter has no incentive to go to sleep on her own as long as company is available. However, it may be too much to expect her to make a major change in one go. The "odd jobs" approach may be your answer. When you have completed your bedtime routine and settled your daughter in her bed, tell her that Mommy and Daddy have things to do in another room. (Be specific: tell her the kitchen, the laundry room, or any room you choose.) Explain that you will listen out for her and that you'll be back in just 5 minutes. If she's upset at this plan, put a clock in her room and show her where the hands will be or what the numbers will say when it's time for you to come back. Leave the room and return in 5 minutes—no more, no less. If she cries or calls for you, answer from outside her room, but don't go back in until the 5 minutes are up. When you go back, praise her for staying in bed, cuddle her if you like, but don't let her get out of bed. Then leave again on another errand, for perhaps a little longer. Make this your practice for the next several nights. Find increasingly time-consuming tasks to do in another room, but always go back briefly to your daughter's bedroom at the time you promised, even if you think she's asleep. She may resist your leaving the first few times. But as she becomes confident that you will return, she will relax, get drowsy, and eventually fall asleep.

she is still learning to be dry at night. Perhaps give her a small drink of water if it's something she needs to settle down.

With bedtime activities, as with other aspects of behavior such as eating and toilet training, let your child take the initiative. If she suggests a reasonable change in the routine, you've nothing to gain by insisting on doing things your way. Your job is to monitor events, making sure that any changes are in the direction of calming rather than stimulating, and keep an eye on the clock. You are there to advise and monitor, occasionally to consent, and now and again to veto. Be consistent, but know when and how to be flexible.

Setting Limits

Children are less likely to develop problems of resistance when their parents set appropriate but firm limits. This applies to going to bed just as it does to other areas of behavior. Enjoy your evening playtime with your child, but bring it to an end when bedtime rolls around. As you get closer to bedtime, activities should be aimed toward preparing your child for bedtime. They should follow a predictable pattern (for example, take a bath, put on pajamas, brush teeth, read a book) and should not consist of activities that will be stimulating (so no television, video games, or active games). With a regular and predictable schedule, your child will be ready for sleep by bedtime.

Make it a general rule that once it's time for sleep, she's to stay in bed until morning. Of course, you must make exceptions and allow your child out when she needs a change or cleanup, comfort after a bad dream, or attention for symptoms such as a fever or vomiting. There is an occasional time, particularly when your child gets older, when she may not be quite sleepy at betime. It is fine to let her have a favorite toy or book to pass the time in her bed. However, no scary stories, television, or video games should be allowed.

GAGGING AND THROWING UP: PROVEN SCARE TACTICS

My son, age 2½, has always gone to sleep with mom or dad lying beside him. Now we're trying to break the habit and get him to go to bed by himself. The problem is, he cries to the point of gagging and almost throws up. Help!

We don't recommend that you leave your toddler to cry until he's too worked up to sleep. However, gagging and throwing up are not harmful in themselves, and some toddlers deliberately gag and make vomiting sounds because they know it's a shortcut to parental attention. A few episodes of minor gagging and throwing up may be an inconvenience you have to put up with to help your child reach the important goal of settling by himself.

Keep this necessary transition period less upsetting for your child by following a regular bedtime routine. Try the "odd jobs" method of gradual withdrawal (see page 76), or sit quietly in your child's room or in a chair just outside the door, where he can still see you as he becomes sleepy. You may have to follow the same procedure several nights in a row, perhaps moving your chair farther from your child's bed and closer to the door (see Chapter 4, "Vanishing Chair Routine," on page 62) until the new habit becomes an established one.

FINDING COMFORT

Toddlers suck their thumbs and cuddle transitional objects—soft toys, blankets—to comfort themselves as they fall asleep. In time, merely sucking the thumb or holding the object may be enough to soothe a child into a drowsy state. A child who can "find" her thumb or fingers to suck will soon lull herself to sleep.

If your infant is fretful at bedtime, a pacifier may help. However, if you use a pacifier, be prepared to have to get up when it falls out of your baby's mouth and she can't find it on her own. You will have to act as a willing retriever until your baby has the coordination to feel for it and put it back in her mouth. Some parents find that putting more than one pacifier in the crib is helpful. Others find that this makes the situation worse because once the child has found a pacifier, she is fully awake and cannot go back to sleep. No matter how many times you have to rescue the pacifier, the American Academy of Pediatrics warns

Do not attempt to solve this problem by tying a pacifier to your child's crib or around your child's neck or hand. This is very dangerous and could cause serious injury or even death.

Early Childhood: When Does a Routine Begin?

It's never too soon to begin developing a going-to-bed routine. From the time your baby is first born, it's good to establish a rhythm. During daylight hours, enjoy increasingly longer periods of wakefulness, talk, and play, and bring the day to a close with a nightly ritual: Wash your baby's face, hands, and bottom; change him into sleep clothes; brush his hair; and rock or cuddle him while singing or listening to quiet music before placing him, still awake but drowsy, in his crib.

Even though your baby may awake for a feeding only a few hours later and will continue to wake up for night feedings for some time, this rhythm helps him to learn that daytime is for waking and nighttime for sleeping. The way you feed him reinforces the message: daytime feedings in bright light, followed by play, then a nap; nighttime feedings in dim light, ending with a prompt return to the crib in a darkened room.

Starting at about 8 weeks, your baby may enjoy listening and watching as you describe what's going on in a picture book. At this age, he is far from being able to follow a story, but you both will enjoy the shared closeness. In this way, you prepare for story reading later on and begin to help your child develop the priceless habit of paying attention.

Crying Before Sleep

For some babies, crying seems to be a way to work off energy as they settle down to sleep and a means of becoming fully alert when they awake. A baby who cries when her parents leave the bedroom may just be saying good night. Left to cry it out, she won't continue wailing for hours. Instead, she'll probably cry and fuss for a few minutes, then soothe herself with a finger or pacifier, and drift into sleep. If she does keep on fussing, the best way to deal with it is to pop your head in the doorway every 5 minutes or so and quietly repeat your usual sign-off, be it "Good night" or "Sleep tight." This lets your baby know that you're nearby but that fun and games are over—it's time to go to sleep. It's important to keep in mind that there are times when you may need to let your baby cry himself to sleep; it won't cause any harm and there's no need to worry about the possible messages behind those tears. Remember, you have all day to show your infant how much you love him and care for him. At night, he'll get the message that nighttime is for sleeping, and on those nights when you let him cry, you're helping him learn to soothe himself. He won't be thinking that you're abandoning him or that you don't love him anymore; he knows by your daytime behaviors that this isn't the case at all. In other words, there's no need to worry.

By the same token, if your baby cries and fusses on waking in the morning, she may not want attention right away. Give her a little while to wake up on her own. She may calm down, sing or babble to herself, and play quietly for a while. Then, if she makes a more insistent cry, take it as a signal that she's ready to get up.

Farther Up the Ladder: Routines in the School Years

For school-aged children, a quick tidy-up is part of the bedtime routine: putting books and toys back on shelves and clothes in drawers and closets. Their room doesn't have to be perfect, but it's more pleasant to rest and read or listen to music and stories in a tidy environment, and mornings go more smoothly if needed objects are where they belong and thus easy to find.

By the middle-school years, the weekend routine is a bit less regimented than the one for school nights, and weekend bedtimes can be later. Lights can go out at different times for different children in the family, depending on how much sleep they need. However, while your child may sleep late the next morning, try to keep weekend wake-ups within an hour or

---

SEPARATION MAY BE MORE STRESSFUL FOR FIRSTBORNS

Problems with separation anxiety tend to loom larger with firstborn and only children. The greater frequency and intensity are often blamed on parents' overeagerness to do the right thing mingled with worry over their inexperience. However, there's another side to the story. First and only children tend to suffer more intense separation anxiety because they feel themselves to be part of a unit with the parents. It's only natural to be frightened of separations that threaten to break up that unit. In a child's mind, going to sleep is one such separation.

When a second child appears on the scene, it's often easier for the first one to understand his place in the family and develop notions of activities and behaviors that are appropriate for children versus adults. And second and later-born children usually—but not always—have less intense anxiety about separation because they are bolstered by the constant presence of the older sibling. (Also see "Sleep and Temperament" on page 82.)

so of the usual time, especially if your child is not a creature of habit by nature. Left to sleep too long, in only a few days a vulnerable child can shift his sleep phase (periods of waking and sleeping) in such a way that he has trouble getting back on his usual schedule. School performance may suffer because he is drowsy when awoken on school days.

SLEEP DIARY

When bedtime refusals or other sleep problems persist despite treatment efforts, including a consistent going-to-bed routine, it's helpful to keep a sleep diary for a week or two. Some pediatricians ask parents to keep a sleep diary as an aid to the diagnosis of sleep problems. Parents use the diary to jot down daily answers to the following questions:

- What did we do during our bedtime routine?
- How long did the bedtime routine last?
- What time did the child actually get into bed and settle down to sleep?
- How long did she cry after the parents left the room?
- How many "curtain calls" (requests for drinks, extra hugs, toilet use) were there before settling?
- How many times did the child awake during the night?
- What steps did the parents take to deal with waking and curtain calls? What time did the child wake up?
- How difficult was it to wake up in the morning?
- Any napping during the day?

A sleep diary helps parents and their child's pediatrician pinpoint aspects of behavior that need attention. It also helps to identify minor problems that are likely to fade away if left alone.

NO MORE "JUST ONE MORE"

A parent who spends the day apart from his child is a soft target for pleas of "just one more" story, game, or other nighttime activity. As with settling a fussy, crying baby, the going-to-bed routine for older children may work more smoothly if the parent who is less susceptible to pressure takes charge.

Keeping Routines Manageable

Unless carefully managed, bedtime routines can be drawn out almost indefinitely, thus defeating the purpose for which they're intended. A child quickly learns that by taking charge of the show, he can significantly delay the time of going to bed. For example, he may have to repeatedly switch his stuffed animals because he can't find quite the right combination to make him sleepy on a particular night. Or he may desperately need the answers to questions that will keep him awake if he has to wait until morning.

Allow your child flexibility within the routine, but keep things under your control by limiting the choices available. For example, let him choose different stuffed animals for bed each night, but keep him to a fixed number. Let him choose a story and a song, but not a whole book or CD. Try to keep the bedtime routine to no longer than 30 minutes.

As your child gets older, you should gradually begin to step back and let him become more in charge of his bedtime routine. Providing these opportunities during his daily routine is also a way to help him become more self-reliant.

Sleep and Temperament

Temperament, or behavioral style, is among the most important factors in determining how children and parents will react in a given situation and how parents teach and care for their children. A baby's basic temperament—easygoing or touchy, calm or irritable—usually begins to be evident in the first weeks of life. It strongly influences the way a caregiver looks after the baby. It also has a major bearing on the way the child develops regular routines, including sleep schedules. Despite the vast range of variations in temperament, a true mismatch between child and parent is unusual. And although definitive studies have not been done, mismatches among adoptive parents and their children appear to be no more frequent than mismatches among biological parents and their offspring.

Although the seeds of temperament are in our genes, temperament is not a fixed characteristic, as gender is. It is modified by many influences in the environment. Some inborn aspects of temperament may take years to emerge, as do certain other genetic traits that are activated in stages. With time, children learn to fit into society by modifying the temperamental characteristics that affect their relationships with others. For example, a naturally shy child may work to overcome his reticence.

Temperament influences the way sleep habits are organized and maintained through a 3-way effect on interactions between the child and his parents or caregivers. First, it affects the way the parent responds to the child's demands. Second, it affects the impact of environmental factors on the child. And third, it affects the way the child responds to the care provided. One sleep expert has noted, "It is often difficult to determine whether disturbed sleep was caused initially by a specific temperament trait or by a parent's behavior…because interactive effects always evolve."

Temperamental interactions may cause many different sleep problems. For instance, parents who try to meet their child's every need may unwittingly set up a vicious cycle of night waking and crying in a child with an intense, irritable temperament. And a child who is naturally persistent may regularly delay bedtime to unreasonable lengths if his parents don't know how to say "No" (see "Keeping Routines Manageable" on page 82). Regardless of the specifics of the case, the result is always the same: The child doesn't get enough sleep, is inattentive and learns poorly at school, and develops a stress response that makes him over-aroused, more difficult, and more emotional.

If this sounds like a problem that may be growing in your family, ask your pediatrician for an impartial evaluation of the situation. Referral to a family therapist may be helpful, and your pediatrician may be able to put you in touch with a support group for parents and children with similar problems.

While misunderstandings can occur in any family, true temperamental mismatches, giving rise to constant conflict, are rare. Successful families are those whose members appreciate and respect one another's temperamental differences and do their best to get along with one another.

DRAW THE LINE

Our 3-year-old son refuses to sleep alone and instead goes to bed with me and my husband between 9:30 and 10:00 pm most nights. He refuses to fall asleep, keeps telling me he wants to play, wants me to get up and watch television with him, and often yells until our ears are ringing that he does not want lights out. This is hard because I need to get up at 5:00 am to be at work by 7:00 am. My son also refuses to take scheduled naps; he only naps when his eyes literally close. If his sitter tries to put him to bed during the day, he screams that he doesn't want to nap, he wants to play. Our 6-year-old daughter has no problem going to her own bed on time at 8:00 pm, but in the middle of the night she also squeezes in with the rest of us. How can we help our children sleep on their own?

Children are happiest when they know who's in charge and what their limits are. Your son, at 3, is far too young to know what's best for him or the family; however, because he's unsure of how far he can go, he constantly tests the boundaries. It's time to lay down some rules and enforce them. You and your husband must agree on a plan and keep to it. In doing so, you will not only help your children to sleep better, but you will also teach them to consider other people's needs and feelings. Unless you do this, your son may have a difficult time getting on with playmates, adjusting to school, and eventually, dealing with life in the wide world.

First, tell your children that from now on, everybody sleeps in his or her own bed. This will let all the family get the sleep they need to work and have fun in the daytime. When your children get up at night, stay calm and lead them back to their own beds. Remember, your son will welcome even negative attention as a reward, so don't get upset—silently count to 10 if it helps—and keep your interaction with him on a low and unemotional level.

Second, set up new rules for television watching, video games, and computer time, allowing a maximum of 1 to 2 hours a day total for all screen time, and in the daytime only. Select the programs your children watch, filter out violent shows and games, and choose materials suitable for your children's age group. Move the television to an inconvenient location if necessary to enforce the new policy. If your child has a television in his bedroom, move it to a different room. Remove any devices that allow him to turn the television on by himself.

Third, when your son wants to play at night, tell him it's not playtime, it's sleep time. Let him have a book and 1 or 2 soft toys to play with quietly in his bed. Leave a night-light in his room and try the "odd jobs" method (see "'Odd Jobs' to Foster Independent Sleeping" on page 76) to keep him in his room. (Make sure that your child's room is childproof—free of breakable or hazardous objects.)

DRAW THE LINE, CONTINUED

In making these changes, you may endure several nights of noise and disruption, but if you are calm and consistent, your children will follow the new rules and your whole family will enjoy better sleep and a more pleasant and restful atmosphere.

Finally, don't be afraid to set limits; your children are asking for them. Your pediatrician may provide information about parent-effectiveness training; many schools, churches, and temples sponsor such programs for developing parenting skills.

COMMONSENSE GUIDELINES FOR SETTLING DOWN AT BEDTIME	
Don't	**Do**
• Let your baby fall asleep at the breast or bottle.	• Place your child in her crib or bed sleepy but still awake.
• Leave your baby with a bottle in bed; this practice can promote ear infections and tooth decay.	• Finish bottle-feeding out of bed.
• Roughhouse in the hour before bedtime.	• Play gently.
• Tell scary or sad stories.	• Read cheerful stories with happy endings.
• Allow screen time in the hour before bedtime.	• Turn off TV, video games, and computers; sing or play relaxing music.
• Give large drinks and heavy snacks just before bedtime.	• Allow a small drink of water or warm milk or light snacks such as cereal, crackers and cheese, yogurt, or fruit. Brush teeth before settling down for the night.
• Rush into your child's room at the first sound you hear.	• Unless you hear a cry of real distress, give your child a few minutes to settle back to sleep on her own.

MANAGING DIFFICULT BEHAVIORS

Although individual cases require specific measures, pediatricians recommend a few general strategies to help parents and children overcome challenging behaviors.

1. Be calm and even-tempered when dealing with your child. Make an effort not to respond emotionally and instinctively, which is usually unproductive.

2. Try not to take your child's behavior personally. Many of the characteristics you find upsetting are inborn; he is not deliberately being annoying. Avoid blaming him or yourself.

3. Set priorities on the issues affecting your child. Deal with the most pressing ones first, then with the rest in order; some may disappear before you get around to them.

4. Deal with problems in the present moment; avoid "What ifs?" and try not to look far into the future.

5. Take an objective look at your own temperament and behavior and try to put yourself in your child's shoes. Perhaps you could find ways to adjust your style to foster a better fit with your child.

6. Anticipate situations in which conflict is likely to occur and try to head them off or keep the impact to a minimum. When problems can't be avoided altogether, accept the possibility that the day may be difficult and be prepared to make the best of it.

7. Ask yourself whether your expectations for your child are realistic. Take every opportunity to praise him for tasks he does right and reinforce the behaviors that you like.

Sleep Disturbances After Separation or Divorce

Each year, more than 1 million children in the United States experience the divorce of their parents. For these children, it can be difficult to maintain consistent bedtimes and going-to-bed routines when they divide their time between 2 homes after a separation or divorce. When custody involves regular weekend and holiday visits to the noncustodial parent, changes in routine are usually taken in stride like other exceptions to a basic schedule. However, in an inherently stressful situation, a child may regress to more babyish or childish behavior, at least for a while. Thumb-sucking and bed-wetting may recur or appear for the first time in a preschooler or school-aged child; night fears may make it hard to settle for sleep. An older child or adolescent may act withdrawn, defiant, or overeager to please. Sleep disturbances—insomnia or oversleeping—are common in children under emotional stress.

Keeping a Consistent Bedtime Routine in 2 Homes

Problems tend to be more difficult to deal with when a child is required to make frequent changes, perhaps spending a few days of the week at one parent's home and the rest at the other's. Sleep disorders, with bedtime refusals and nighttime waking, are common among children who feel torn between 2 parents, 2 homes, and 2 different routines.

Problems may arise out of conflict due to widely different styles in the 2 homes, regardless of the custody arrangements. In an extreme case, a perfectionist parent who allows no flexibility at all in schedules for meals and bedtimes may be pitched against the former partner, who lets the children snack without restraint and go to sleep where they drop in front of the television. A person would have to be an emotional quick-change artist to make such a demanding about-face every few days. Yet many children are asked to do just that; the child has no sooner adapted to one home when she must adjust to the other. Difficulties arise out of irregularity in routines and lack of cooperation between parents. To help ease the situation, keep duplicates of especially favorite bedtime toys, books, or music at both homes to prevent problems due to haste or forgetfulness.

When parents work together, it makes the transition easier for the child. It takes unusually close teamwork between the 2 parents to make an arrangement work—perhaps even closer than when they lived under one roof. Once the family's situation has stabilized, sleep problems and other symptoms should gradually disappear over several weeks. If they persist, talk to your pediatrician, who may suggest a referral for counseling and possibly participation in a support group.

Keep Communication Channels Open

Children tend to have more frequent sleep disturbances after their parents separate or divorce. In young children, this increase is due to a surge in separation anxiety stemming from fear of abandonment by both parents. "After all," the child may reason, "if one parent has left our home for good, what's to keep the other from doing the same?"

Whether you're the custodial or noncustodial parent, each time you leave your child in the care of another person, let him know when you'll be back or when you expect to speak with him next: "I'll pick you up next Friday at 6:00," or "Call me before you leave for school

tomorrow." If you don't know the exact time, give a guideline: "I'll be home in time for dinner," or "I'll be back tonight but not until after you're in bed, so let's talk tomorrow morning."

Remember that children can deal with disappointing news, but lack of information worries
them and stimulates their imagination. Indeed, the fewer facts they have to work with, the
more elaborate their imaginary explanations are likely to be. Left to figure situations out for
themselves, children tend to fear the worst.

Here are recommendations from the American Academy of Pediatrics about talking with
your child early and often.

- Be completely honest and open about what is happening. The more you're talking, the
  more comfortable your child will feel.
- Make sure your child knows the divorce is not his fault.
- Try not to blame your ex-spouse or show your anger.
- Be patient with questions. Your child may ask, "Why are you getting divorced?" or "Are
  you ever going to get back together?"

Night Owls

Young Children

There are children—even toddlers and preschoolers—who take a long time to get to sleep
after a regular going-to-bed routine, despite their own and their parents' best efforts. In
almost all cases, these children also wake up later in the morning, are hard to rouse, and
tend to be cranky for some time after waking. Some of these children are true night owls
(they were born with a preference for a later schedule); however, most have just become
used to a later schedule. This occurs when, for whatever reason, the child's sleep schedule
gets later and later, and because there is no effort to keep the schedule consistent, the wake
times also get later and later.

If your child is one of these who does not want to fall asleep, you first need to make sure
that you wake him up at a consistent time every morning (even weekends). If the usual and
target wake times are far apart, you may have to do this over a few days. He will probably be

cranky and will be tired during the course of the day. Then you can begin to slowly make his bedtime earlier and earlier until you get to the target bedtime (see "Suggested Schedule for Reprogramming a Late Sleeper" below). Controlling light exposure also helps to reset the child's internal clock. Turn on lights and open the window shades 1 to 2 hours before the target wake time. You can also dim lights and turn off the television and video games as the target bedtime approaches.

SUGGESTED SCHEDULE FOR REPROGRAMMING A LATE SLEEPER	
Nights	**Bedtimes**
1–2	10:00 pm
3–5	9:45 pm
6–8	9:30 pm
9–11	9:15 pm
12–14	9:00 pm
15–17	8:45 pm
18–20	8:30 pm
21–23	8:15 pm
24–26	8:00 pm

WAKING TOO EARLY

My 5-year-old gets up too early. His bedtime is 9:00 pm (changed from 8:00 pm in an effort to delay his waking) and he wakes up between 4:00 and 5:00 am. By noon he's tired out. Unfortunately, he was assigned to a kindergarten class that begins at 12:30 pm. He's irritable, sometimes behaves disruptively, and usually wants to take a nap in the middle of class. We've installed dark shades in his room (it's still dark when he wakes, anyway) and we don't know what else to do. Should we keep him up even later?

Your child's schedule and circadian rhythm don't match, and he is trying to compensate for this by taking a nap at school. Keep a consistent bedtime routine, but begin moving his bedtime later by 15 minutes every 1 to 2 nights until you reach the point when he is beginning to sleep later in the morning. In the meantime, try to give him quiet activities to do in the morning so that he is not worn out by noon.

If you follow this schedule consistently for several weeks, your son's sleep phase (the hours out of 24 in a day he spends asleep) should shift so that he is waking later in the morning. If this does not work, consulting a sleep specialist may be helpful.

LARKS (EARLY WAKERS) VERSUS OWLS (LATE SLEEPERS)

The differences between so-called *larks* and *owls* involve more than just times for getting up and going to bed. Thanks to the circadian rhythms governing hormone secretion and temperature regulation, owls are always at their best and most alert late in the evening and always have trouble getting up and on the go in the morning, no matter how long they have slept. And for larks, of course, the opposite is true. However, although very early waking can be a problem with young children, few parents worry about a lark who goes to sleep at a reasonable hour and wakes up bright-eyed and ready for action.

If you have an owl-child in your family, he may find it difficult to fall asleep at the bedtime you've set, even when you keep to a strict schedule. Luckily, although many adults fall into this pattern, children are somewhat more adaptable.

It's important to maintain an owl on the same daily schedule for waking, even on weekends, to prevent the circadian rhythms from shifting steadily later. Keep your child's bedtime routines calm and unhurried, and let sleep associations induce a feeling of relaxation leading to drowsiness.

Shifting the Sleep Phase

One way to solve your late sleeper's problem may be to shift his sleep phase (see Chapter 9, Adolescence: Ages 13+) so that he feels tired and goes to sleep earlier. However, shifting the sleep phase is not always easy, and it cannot be done in a single step. If you put your child to bed at 7:00 pm when he is used to falling asleep at 10:00 pm, he will have to endure hours of wakefulness and possibly boredom. This is unlikely to make him enjoy being in bed; instead, he may view his bed as a place of punishment rather than a comfortable refuge.

It's better to use a gradual approach. Start with the time your child wakes up as your baseline and work back with a quarter-hour change about every 3 or 4 days until your child has reprogrammed his pattern and is now sleepy at the bedtime you want. For example, if he regularly drops off at 10:00 pm and wakes up at 8:00 am, start your new schedule by waking him up for the first day or two at 7:45 am. Then, for the next 3 or 4 days, wake him up at 7:30 am. By the final night, he should be adjusted to getting sleepy at the new time. Continue the reprogramming with a 15-minute change every 3 or 4 days until your child is ready for bed at your target bedtime. One month is usually long enough for the adjustment. If you hit a snag at any quarter-hour stage during the process, don't give up or go back. Spend a few more days at the latest level that was reached, then restart the process with that time as your new baseline.

Remember that wake-up time is more important than bedtime in shifting the sleep phase and regulating circadian rhythms. Once you adjust your child's schedule, keep to a single wake-up time and do not vary it, even on weekends. Bright light in the morning can also help maintain wake time.

Vacations and Sleepovers

The key to having the whole family sleep well on vacations is to temper the novelty of a new environment with some of the familiar sensations that your child finds comforting. Of course, you wouldn't leave home without teddy or ducky, or whoever the favorite bedtime companion may be. You may also play it safe by taking the blanket and pillow your child is used to. But even if your child is an infant, don't underestimate her willingness to get into the vacation spirit and enjoy a change of surroundings. A child who is used to a regular routine at home generally adapts well to change because she remains confident that her needs will be met, no matter where she finds herself.

Whatever your child's age may be, try to keep her on her normal sleep/wake schedule during vacations. If the vacation involves travel to a different time zone, adopt local time from the moment you arrive, but be prepared to allow for naps at odd times to make up for sudden onsets of fatigue. As soon as you get home, switch back immediately to your regular time. Children are adaptable. Once your child gets back to her usual schedule for play, meals, and sleep, any disturbance in her sleep/wake cycle will probably disappear within a few days. It generally takes about 1 day to adjust to each hour of time change; so, for instance, if you are travelling to somewhere that is 3 hours behind where you live, you can anticipate that it will take about 3 days to adjust when you get there and another 3 days to adjust back when you return.

Staying Up Late

On special holidays and family celebrations, even the youngest members of the family get to stay up late. This means they may miss out on the usual bedtime routine. A child who stays up way past bedtime may become overtired and grouchy after a day full of fun. In this frame of mind she may have trouble relaxing for sleep. A shortened version of your bedtime routine—one song, one story, one animal to hug—may do the trick.

Lots of family outings end with children falling asleep in the car on the way home and being carried to bed without waking. Children often sleep better if you anticipate these events when possible by washing them, changing them into sleep clothes, and brushing teeth before leaving for home. There are sleep experts who insist that once home, you should wake your child and put him through the usual routine. However, others disagree. Unless you are dealing with a child whose unusually rigid, compulsive personality adapts poorly to change, it's probably not worth waking a sleeping child just to go through the motions of a bedtime routine. Let sleeping dogs and children lie.

Spring Forward, Fall Back

Changes for daylight saving time in the spring and fall may disrupt your child's sleeping patterns for a few days after clocks are reset. When clocks move forward an hour in the spring, bedtime is an hour earlier and your child will still be wide awake. He may take a long time to become drowsy. It is sometimes helpful to gradually change the bedtime over a few days.

Again, when clocks are turned back an hour in the fall, no special measures need be taken. Your child will probably be tired before the clock says it's time for bed. It won't do any harm to let him get ready for bed a little earlier than usual. He may also wake a bit earlier for the first few days but will soon be back on track, provided you follow a regular timetable.

If you run into difficulties on either side of the change, try the 15-minute schedule suggested in "Shifting the Sleep Phase" on page 91. Also, check the light level in your child's bedroom and make any necessary adjustments by installing window coverings or adding an extra lamp. Prolonged light in the evenings may make it hard to fall asleep for some children, just as darkness in the mornings may make it harder to get up.

CHAPTER 6

Twins and More

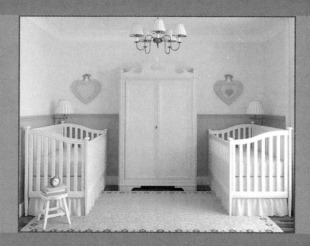

*T*he majority of sleep challenges related specifically to multiple births are faced in the first year of your babies' lives. Sleep becomes easier after the first year.

Multiple births, once rare, now occur quite commonly. The rate of identical twinning, which occurs when 2 children develop from a single fertilized egg, has stayed the same, but the frequency of fraternal (multiple-egg) twins and triplets is soaring, thanks in part to treatments based on the harvesting and fertilization of several eggs at a time. It is not all due to in vitro fertilization, as increased use of fertility treatments (for example, hormones such as clomiphene [Clomid]) are also partly responsible. As a result, the number of multiple births has increased 42% since 1990 and 70% since 1980.

The greater the number of babies born from a single pregnancy, the greater the likelihood that they will be premature and smaller compared with single babies born at term. For that reason, many of the sleep patterns and disruptions seen in twins and multiples are the same as those seen in premature and low birth weight babies (also see Chapter 1, "Sleep Patterns in a Premature Baby," on page 14). In addition, multiple gestation babies are at higher risk for sudden infant death syndrome (SIDS) and other accidental sleep deaths, so it is especially important to follow safe sleep guidelines for the first year of life (see Chapter 2).

When what you expected to be a single baby turns out to be 2 babies, or 3, or more, the potential for sleep problems is doubled or tripled, and so are the challenges in dealing with them. You may be surprised to learn that each of your babies has a different temperament and personality—one of your babies may be a more restful sleeper than her co-twin. Strategies that work for one baby may need to be tweaked for another. Luckily, you can also have twice as much pleasure and sense of accomplishment when situations, such as sleep, are under control. Good sleep habits will only benefit the emotional and physical health of your suddenly expanded family.

Your babies need proper sleep to grow and develop, and just as importantly, you as a parent will need adequate sleep to successfully navigate the challenges of your growing family. No matter how self-reliant you were before your babies arrived on the scene, this is one time when it's truly difficult to go it alone. Don't be afraid to ask for help. Your significant other may need specific guidance as to how to assist with the babies' sleep schedules. A parent's single night of 6 hours of interrupted sleep will allow him to handle the following day much better. Do not assume your partner will instinctively know what needs to be accomplished; good communication is quite important at this stage in your babies' lives. Your family and friends will likely be glad to lend a hand. At the same time, do not hesitate to ask your baby's pediatrician for advice and support more often than if you had given birth to just one baby.

TWO IN A BED

I just found out that the baby we planned is going to be twins. The only room we can set aside is quite small and I don't see how we could fit 2 cribs in it. Would it be all right to have our babies share a crib?

For safety reasons, we recommend that each child have an individual bassinet, crib, or bed. Not only will your babies sleep safer with 2 separate cribs, but they will be more comfortable as well. This also decreases the chance that one baby will catch an infection from the other baby. Sleeping bag pajamas or, when the babies are a bit older, fleeced footed pajamas would be preferable to blankets and covers for keeping the babies warm; keep soft quilts as well as stuffed animals out of your babies' sleeping space to avoid risk of sudden infant death syndrome.

Perhaps, in the time before your twins are born, you may be able to reconfigure the space you've set aside. For example, it may be possible to gain space by using part of a hallway or a closet with the door removed. You can also consider using portable cribs or play yards while the babies are small, as these take up less space. If the cribs are placed side by side or end to end where your babies can see each other, they will thrive on each other's company on waking and going to sleep.

Remember that any crib you use needs to meet the new safety standards from the US Consumer Product Safety Commission (CPSC) that went into effect in June 2011. Under these new rules, all cribs manufactured and sold in the United States must comply with the safety rules, which prohibit the use of cribs that have drop-side rails and strengthen crib slats and mattress supports. For more information, go to the CPSC Web site, www.cpsc.gov.

Where Do We Start?

The first goal after you bring your twins or multiples home is to get them onto the same schedule for feeding, playing, bathing, dressing, and—above all—sleeping. While this is not medically necessary, it certainly will make life logistically easier for you. Newborns often require about 14 to 16 hours of sleep in a 24-hour period, broken up into smaller naps through the day and evening. Because feeding and sleeping are the 2 primary activities of newborns, as a parent you can use sleeping and feeding to coordinate the babies' schedules.

Here are general guidelines on the amount of sleep that your infant requires at 2 to 3 months of age.

- Nighttime sleep should last for about 9 to 10 hours. However, don't expect these 9 to 10 hours to be uninterrupted sleep!
- The remainder of baby's sleep time—about 5 hours—should be divided up into 3 naps during the day.

As you've already read, your multiples may have been born prematurely and they may be smaller than the average term baby, so they may need to be fed during the night for a longer time. But as they gain more weight, they'll eventually sleep through the night on their own, meaning that they sleep for more than 5 to 6 hours at a time. All babies eventually do. Once your multiples weigh about 12 pounds, their stomach capacities will have increased, and they'll outgrow the need for those middle-of-the-night feedings.

Initially, babies can usually only tolerate being awake for 90 minutes or so. Because they may have their own temperaments, don't be surprised if twin B always wakes up first, for example. But when one wakes up to eat, awaken both babies to eat. Feed them simultaneously (with the help of a twin-feeding pillow, easily found for purchase online), which simplifies a single caregiver's task of tandem nursing (or bottle-feeding babies together). Try not to feel guilty about always waking up twin A; over time and with consistency, they will both naturally wake up at similar times.

After feeding, the babies will need to be burped and held. Then, following some playtime, tummy time, and a diaper change, soon it will be time for the next nap. Try to keep your multiples on the same schedule for these daily repetitive activities to simplify their care—and to maintain your own sanity.

Your pediatrician can give you additional advice on how to make enough time in the day for everything that needs to be done during each 24-hour cycle. If you create routines, make sure you schedule time for each of the twins (not to mention for your spouse, your other children, and yourself). If you can create bedtime routines when your twins get their sleep, you may actually find you have an extra hour or two to do nothing more than enjoy the new additions to your family. You'll also find that this routine helps you put both babies on the same schedule—napping at the same time and eating together. A schedule can also help you conserve your own energy and reduce your risk of feeling depleted much of the time.

As your babies continue to grow, take opportunities to communicate to them that nighttime is for sleeping. Keep the lights dimmed when you go to a crib to change a diaper. Until they no longer need nighttime feedings, do so with as little commotion as possible, and then leave the crib so they can return to sleep . By about 9 months of age, your babies will develop what's called *object permanence,* meaning that they recognize that you still exist even when you're not in their line of sight, which makes it easier for them to get back to sleep when you leave their room.

It is particularly challenging for parents of more than one baby to find time to sleep themselves. Consider enlisting the aid of a reliable caregiver, including quality sitters, for a few hours a day, and take a nap while you have someone else keeping an eye on the babies. Friends and relatives are often pleased to help out. Several parents of multiples have been kept afloat in the early months by rosters of volunteer helpers from their churches, temples, and local service organizations. When someone offers assistance, don't be bashful; ask, "When can you come?" Keep a calendar for signing up helpers and call to confirm scheduled appointments; otherwise you may find yourself with more help than you need one day and on your own the next. Eventually, as the babies settle into a regular routine and learn to self-soothe, fewer extra hands will be needed.

Who's on First?

A common fear of parents of twins is that when one child starts crying, the other will follow suit. There's a tendency, therefore, to rush into the bedroom at the first whimper and placate baby A with a picking up or a feeding to keep him quiet and thus avoid waking baby B. The risk is that by responding too quickly, you may foster a sleep/wake problem if one infant tends to cry more than the other. If you pick him up to soothe him or offer an unscheduled and unnecessary feeding, he may develop a habit of waking at the same time every night.

Surprisingly, many twins and multiples *don't* wake each other up with their crying, at least not in the first year or so. Most of the time, one baby will sleep through the other's crying—perhaps only to wake up for his turn as soon as the first has settled down. When you have more than 2 babies, however, the chances of at least 2 babies waking up at the same time are much greater. Once the night-feeding phase is over, nighttime waking in multiples is best handled as recommended for single children (see Chapter 1).

If one or more babies needs a clean diaper, attend to the change with the least possible disturbance. Keep the room dim, speak softly and only as much as you have to, change the diaper in the crib if you can, and if you have to take him out of the crib, put the baby right back in the crib when you're finished. When everybody's needs have been attended to, quickly turn out the lights so that the babies know it's time to go back to sleep. A white noise machine or a fan directed at a wall can muffle outside noises as well as signal that it is sleeping time.

What if a baby is healthy, older than 3 months, and weighs more than 12 pounds—and he keeps on crying for longer than a few minutes after you turn out the lights? First of all, for a non-multiple, 5 to 10 minutes of crying is considered a general acceptable guideline, but with multiple babies you may want to wait a shorter time if you are concerned about disturbing the other. Then, when time is up for that crying baby, go to him without turning on the light, pat his back or rub him gently, and quietly tell him it's time to sleep, then leave again (also see Chapter 3). Repeat your visits as necessary, but be firm: no picking up. On the other hand, if a preemie is underweight and due for a feeding, then you (or the caregiver) must absolutely feed him.

When more than one baby is awake and crying (unless you've intentionally awakened one of them so both can eat together), it may be too much for one person to handle. As we've already pointed out, occasionally parents are in a position to employ caregivers, including for nighttime care. Other lucky families have a grandparent or other relative who has the time and inclination to lend a hand. In most families, however, parents eventually have to find the best way to manage on their own. This is no time for one parent to hold back with "It's your turn, I went last time." Both have to pitch in. This exhausting phase will pass, and good communication and a cooperative attitude will make it much easier.

PEAS IN A POD

One mother was concerned about promoting the individual identities of her twin daughters. She took pains never to dress the identical girls in similar outfits. She cut their hair differently and, when they were past the toddler stage, encouraged separate friendships and play dates. Going to bed alone and learning self-soothing skills alone were part of the individualized approach. At age 5, the girls enjoyed their independence in most aspects but begged and pleaded until their parents agreed to put their twin beds in a single room.

All Together Now…or Separate But Equal?

One question you'll have to address after the first few months is whether your twins or multiples will have separate bedrooms (space in your home permitting) or share a room. There are 2 schools of thought on this issue. Parents firmly on the side of separate rooms prefer that their multiples get used to seeing themselves as individuals right from the start. Such parents generally try to maintain a "separate but equal" policy in all aspects of their children's care.

The difficulty with this method is that even though the children are on the same schedule, you may have to stagger bedtimes somewhat. One solution is to alternate the rooms in which the nighttime routine takes place. If both parents are always available at bedtime, they may split the work to give each baby some one-on-one attention. Or perhaps a child care helper can pitch in at bedtime. Many families with multiples enjoy a bedtime routine that includes one-on-one time with the caregiver, who spends time with each twin individually reading children's picture books in separate rooms of the house (it doesn't have to be in the bedroom; you can even use the main family living area). This practice not only fosters

---

TWO BY TWO

My twins are due 3 months from now and I'm already losing sleep worrying about how I'm going to juggle 2 babies when they wake up for nighttime feedings. Do I feed one, then the other? What happens if they both cry at the same time?

Feeding twins requires some special strategies. Now is a good time to talk with your pediatrician, who will be able to guide and reassure you with some useful advice about night feedings in new-born twins. Your pediatrician may also suggest that you get in touch with a lactation consultant—a specially trained nurse or other health care professional—who is experienced in helping mothers of multiple births prepare for breastfeeding. To make it easier, a mother is sometimes advised to express human milk and have her partner bottle-feed one baby while she breastfeeds the other. In this way, the babies take turns at the breast and Dad has an opportunity to share in nighttime care. Be prepared, but take the lead from your babies and don't anticipate problems. When the time comes, you'll manage beautifully.

Raising Twins: From Pregnancy to Preschool by Shelly Vaziri Flais, MD, FAAP, is a resource you may want to read during pregnancy to prepare for your bundles of joy.

---

emotional family bonds but helps each child's self-esteem and burgeoning identity, all the while boosting literacy.

After early infancy, however, story time and other bedtime routines and rituals (also see Chapter 5) for both children can be combined to take place in neutral territory, such as the living room; the youngsters can be separated at the moment of actually going to bed. On the other hand, many parents prefer to keep twins and multiples together because as they get to know each other, they know that they can help comfort one another instead of demanding a parent.

Sometimes, once babies get used to one another's company (which may happen as early as 4 months of age and certainly will between 6 and 9 months), they may cry for each other and refuse to be parted at night. Even if they have slept separately until now, they may want to share a room for at least a year or two. Far better to follow their lead and have them sleep contentedly with 2 cribs or beds in 1 room than to insist on separate rooms before they are ready.

By the way, twins sharing a bedroom tends to lead to some unique and wonderful experiences only shared by other parents of twins sharing a bedroom. At bedtime, when parents say good night and the door is closed, older twin babies (7 to 10 months, for example), will often babble and "talk" with one another, using their early forms of communication. The sounds of your twins or multiples chatting with one another, even at such a young age, is an incredible and priceless feeling—and well-earned with all your hard work!

YOU'LL NEVER WALK ALONE...
Twins and multiples go through phases of night waking, just as singletons do. However, although there are few scientific studies on separation anxiety in children of multiple births, parents of twins and multiples claim informally that their children—like later-born children—seem to be less troubled by separation anxiety than singletons, especially firstborn single children.

Musical Chairs

More often than not, parents of multiples have fewer bedrooms than children. If the children are spread out over 2 or 3 bedrooms, it may be an idea to switch beds every few months so the children can enjoy a change of nighttime company and you can also determine the best combinations to ensure peaceful nights for everyone. Two particular children together, for example, may excite each other but may stay calmer if they are split up to share bedrooms with other siblings, whether identical in age or older members of the family.

A Few Words About Bunk Beds

Children love bunk beds, but they can be dangerous. The child in the top bunk can fall out, and the child in the lower bunk can be injured if the upper bunk collapses. If you accept these risks and decide to install bunk beds anyway, take the following precautions to keep your child safe:

1. Do not allow a child younger than 6 years to sleep in the top bunk. A child younger than 6 years does not have the coordination to climb safely or to keep from falling out.

2. Place bunk beds in a corner, with walls on 2 sides. This not only helps to brace the beds but also eliminates 2 out of the 4 possible sides where a child could fall out of bed.

3. Make sure the top mattress fits snugly within the frame and cannot ride over the edge.

4. Attach a ladder to the top bunk. Place a night-light so your child can see the ladder.

5. Install a guardrail on the top bunk, with a space no wider than 3½ inches between the guardrail and the side of the bunk. Check to make sure your child can't roll under the guardrail when the mattress is pressed down by the weight of his body. Replace the mattress or place a thick pad under the old mattress if necessary.

6. Check that the mattress is supported by wires or slats that run directly underneath and are fastened in place at both ends. A mattress held up only by the bed frame or unsecured slats could fall through to the lower bunk.

7. If you separate the bunks into twin beds, remove all dowels and connectors.

8. To stop children from falling and avoid weakening the structure, do not allow children to jump or roughhouse on either bunk.

THOUGHTS ABOUT TODDLERS

Toddler and preschooler twins will give up their daytime naps sooner compared with singletons. You may need to do some creative trial-and-error so they do not disturb each other if one continues napping for longer than the other. Perhaps one child can sleep in his usual shared bedroom and the other in a sibling's or parent's bedroom so they do not disturb each other.

Preschool twins—or any child, for that matter—should not give up their naps cold turkey but instead should transition to an hour of quiet time with picture books or a loved stuffed animal (but no television). This may be tricky to enforce and the caregiver may need to be physically present to ensure that the quiet time doesn't turn into playtime (or wrestling time!).

A couple of additional points: As your twins grow, they will learn to climb out of the crib from watching one another. You need to be prepared for that day and should think about placing their crib mattresses on the floor for safety until you can decide whether to buy them toddler beds or twin beds.

As your twins become more mobile and able to crawl out of their cribs and move about the bedroom, install a pressure-mounted gate on the bedroom door. Do this *before* your babies start leaving their cribs. Your priority is to keep them safe in their room at all hours and not let them endanger themselves by roaming loose in the house.

As your twins become older, there will be new challenges all along the way, but they can all be dealt with. Once your twins reach ages 3 and 4 years, they should be sleeping a total of 12 hours in each 24-hour period. They may no longer feel the need for naps (typically around 2½ to 3 years of age) except after nights in which they went to sleep late or awakened early. Sometimes, simply encouraging them to have some quiet time (perhaps an hour or so) at midday will energize them for the rest of the day that lies ahead. If they get lots of exercise and other activity during the day, it will help make sure that they sleep well at night. A cumulative total of 30 minutes a day of activity will make falling asleep at night a little easier. Keep in mind, however, that if they become overtired, they may have more trouble nodding off at bedtime.

If your child has difficulty settling at bedtime, some pediatricians recommend creating a sleep success sticker calendar. In her book *Raising Twins: From Pregnancy to Preschool,* Shelly Vaziri Flais, MD, FAAP, describes the friendly competition between her twins that helped them sleep through the night. The children could keep track of their progress with stickers and a calendar, with the prize of a sticker on a calendar date each time they fell asleep quietly. "After 5 stickers, for example, the child earns a small prize (your local dollar store is a perfect place to choose such a prize). Start with a low number of stickers to earn a prize to give each child a taste of success, and then raise the bar, increasing the number of stickers to earn a prize as your twins learn acceptable sleep behavior....A little friendly competition can be a good thing if it will help everyone sleep through the night again!"

CHAPTER 7

Preschoolers

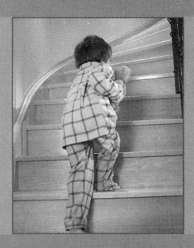

*S*leep deprivation is rare in children younger than school age because most have the ability to fall asleep almost anywhere and at any time to make up for missed day or nighttime sleep. If there's a problem at this age, it's more likely to be one of scheduling: a preschooler who naps too long during the day and then stays awake late at night or whose sleep time is otherwise out of sync with that of the rest of the family.

Your child's typical resistance and moodiness may give way to a period of sweet sensibility at around age 3. In general, however, these preschool years are marked by phases of calm behavior alternating with periods of exploration or opposition. The need to resist adult boundaries with parents and caregivers with daily routines such as eating, dressing, and going to bed allows your preschooler to gauge his position in the family and the degree to which he can control his environment. It's all part of his long drive to become an independent person. To give your child a feeling of control, give him choices to make at bedtime—for example, which pajamas to wear, which books to read, or which stuffed animal to snuggle with in bed.

Most preschool-aged children (3 to 5 years old) are ready for nighttime sleep between 7:00 and 9:00 pm, or earlier if naps are brief or absent, and they'll sleep through the night until about 6:30 to 8:00 am. Naps tend to become less frequent in some children by age 3 or 4.

Preschoolers by and large are busy and active all day long. Most give up their daytime naps as they approach age 5. Some need an earlier bedtime when they first stop napping. They or you can tell when they are ready to give up their afternoon nap when there is difficulty getting them to go to sleep at their usual bedtime. And although most may try resistance or delaying tactics at bedtime, most in the preschool years will sleep for 10 to 12 hours a night. For the great majority of these preschoolers, nighttime waking is uncommon. This is the time, however, when sleep disturbances such as sleepwalking and night terrors (see Chapter 11) are likely to appear in susceptible children.

Rapid Eye Movement Versus Non-Rapid Eye Movement Sleep

At every age, children's sleep patterns are influenced by interactions among developmental, biological, and emotional factors.

During the preschool years, children begin to have recurrent, longer episodes of non-rapid eye movement (REM) (non-dreaming) sleep with partial arousals that occur during the transitions from non-REM to REM phases throughout the night. Non-REM sleep consists of several phases—drowsiness, light sleep, and deep sleep. There is no dreaming during non-REM sleep, and your child is virtually motionless. Conditions known as *parasomnias*—sleepwalking, sleep talking, and night terrors (also see Chapter 11)—are defined as *partial arousals* and are common in this age group. Some children have more frequent episodes of partial arousal when they are overtired or during periods of emotional stress, such as family upheavals or school examinations. Children generally do not remember these episodes in the morning.

OPPOSITE POINTS OF VIEW

My 3-year-old daughter often wakes and cries in the night. After we have calmed her, she stays quiet for a few minutes but then starts crying for us again. My wife wants to let her cry herself back to sleep, but I feel I must go back and calm her. Should we let her cry or is it all right to go back for a few minutes? When she cries, I can't sleep, but my wife says I am setting our daughter up for a lifetime of sleep problems.

What's important is that you and your wife agree on an approach and join forces to put it into practice. Even if you are not setting your daughter up for a lifetime of sleep troubles, you may unintentionally be giving her the message that "divide and conquer" is a sure path to power. In other words, if Mommy says, "No," go ask Daddy. Depending on the maturity level of your child, you may also want to have a discussion with her during daytime hours about how you plan to address the nighttime crying.

Once your preschooler is calm and drowsy again, pat her a couple of times and leave the room. When you keep going back as soon as you hear a whimper, you reinforce her crying, instead of helping her comfort herself and fall asleep. Maybe you and your wife can agree on a back-patting schedule that you both participate in where you slowly reduce the number of times you go into her room.

Nightmares occur during REM sleep, so they are not associated with non-REM partial arousals; children often can describe what happened in the nightmare. Nightmares are common in the preschool years and may also be triggered by emotional trauma and stress.

THREE-YEAR-OLD CHALLENGES

Our 3-year-old still wakes up once or twice most nights. It's almost always because she is cold; she goes to sleep once we pull the covers back over her. We've tried to show her how to pull up her own covers, but she simply refuses to do it. If we don't go in, she yells louder and becomes more awake. She's a fairly well-behaved, obedient child in most other respects. What can we do to get some shut-eye?

Explain to your daughter that although you will always help her if she's sick or something is wrong at night, you can no longer get up just to pull the covers over her. Perhaps you could buy an inexpensive sleeping bag or blanket-sleeper pajamas. Let her sleep in the zipped-up sleeping bag or blanket sleeper until she learns to pull up her own covers.

Your Child's Biological Rhythms

Give some thought to other factors that could play a role in your child's sleep. Have you put her on a timetable that might conflict with her own biological rhythms, or is she in sync with her natural rhythms?

You can help your child sleep better through the timing of her sleep, which can restore alertness and encourage an even temperament. Pay attention to your preschooler and her daily "circadian rhythms" and see if she seems to have drowsy periods. If you encourage her to sleep or rest during those times when she appears drowsy, her sleep patterns are likely to match her internal rhythms. Otherwise, you may be trying to get her to sleep too early or too late for her to achieve fully restorative sleep. Keep in mind that the quality of her sleep depends largely on *when* she sleeps, rather than *how long* she sleeps.

How can you tell if your preschooler is getting enough quality rest? Keep an eye on her at the end of the day, and if she seems friendly, adaptable, and engaging, she's probably sleeping at the right time. But if she becomes hyperactive or irritable, she may be growing weary as the day draws to a close and her sleep deprivation is on the increase.

Other Approaches to Making Sleep Work

As a parent, you will be flooded with advice, whether you ask for it or not, about how to get your preschooler to eat, walk, talk, become potty trained, and sleep. Again, as a parent, you're in the best position to understand your child's needs, according to his temperament.

Thank your friends and relatives for their well-meant suggestions, but take your cues from the one person who knows how to deal with these natural functions: your child. You will soon find ways that suit both of you and that allow him to develop at his own pace. As always, your child's pediatrician can be a great resource.

When bedtime resistance arises in a preschooler, it's often possible to head off trouble by setting up a neutral timekeeper. Put a clock in your child's room, tell him you'll stay with him until "the little hand is on 8 and the big hand is on 9" or "the numbers are 7 4 5" (or whatever

---

OTHER OPINIONS

Friends encourage my partner and me to allow our preschooler to sleep with us. They warn us that our failure to "nighttime parent" will cause our child to be insecure and that our approach—having our child sleep in a separate bed and letting him cry for a while as long as he's not uncomfortable—is inhumane. This method has worked for us; our child sleeps well. Of course, if he awakens during the night and cries persistently, we go in at once to see if anything's wrong. However, I now feel guilty about doing this. Could a method that works so well be wrong in the long run because, as our friends claim, it promotes psychological damage?

Time and again in this book, we emphasize that there are few cut-and-dried solutions to children's sleep problems. The best solution is the one that works for your family.

It sounds as if you have found such a solution: Your child sleeps well and receives as much nighttime parenting as he needs. There is no evidence that the approach you have adopted leads to psychological problems. Thank your friends for their suggestions, chalk them up to differences of parenting opinions, and let it pass.

time you choose), and pace your bedtime routine so that it winds to a close with the clock. You may even want to set an alarm for the start of his bedtime so that there is no question about when bedtime is.

Instead of a clock, your child may prefer starting a kitchen timer for 5-, 10-, and 15-minute intervals. The timekeeper method has a twofold benefit: It's the impartial clock—and not the parent—that says it's time for bed, and it expands your child's understanding of numbers and how they are related to telling time.

There's rarely a single answer to every sleep problem, and different approaches may be needed at various times to help your child overcome a particular obstacle. For example, we advise that children should fall asleep in their own beds. But this guidance is occasionally set aside in many families without lasting disruption. At one time or another, parents may curl up together with a feverish or fearful preschooler and, depending on their age, have no difficulty in returning to the normal routine as soon as the episode of illness or nightmares is passed.

Shutting the Door

It's never acceptable to keep a child's bedroom door locked at night. In case of an emergency, such as a fire, the child cannot get out of a locked bedroom and parents may be unable to unlock the door in time. Moreover, a child who is forcibly kept in his room behind a locked door will not develop the self-control to stay there willingly. And if a resentful child is forced to stay unsupervised in his room, he may injure himself or damage objects in the room. If a child is anxious about being alone or has separation anxiety, it may worsen the situation.

However, when you are dealing with a persistent nighttime rambler, some parents find that the door can be a useful aid. Many children prefer to go to sleep with the bedroom door ajar. Tell your child that as long as he remains in bed, the door can stay open. The moment he gets out of bed, the door will be shut.

If you use a night-light, make sure it is dim and not right by the child's head. Even a light from the bathroom may also be bright enough to be disturbing.

A 4-YEAR-OLD KNOWS WHAT SHE'S USED TO

My daughter, who just had her fourth birthday, will not sleep through the night in her room. She falls asleep in the living room and then we put her into bed. A short time later, she wakes up and wants to go back into the living room.

Your daughter is comfortable in the living room because that is where she's used to falling asleep. The living room has become a sleep association for her, and if she wakes up, she cannot fall asleep again without being in the living room. She will be able to sleep in her bedroom if she learns to fall asleep there.

Establish a consistent bedtime routine for sleep (perhaps stories, hair brushing, putting toys to bed; see other chapters for suggestions, such as Chapter 3, "Preventing Bedtime Resistance," on page 43) that takes place entirely in your daughter's room. If there are playthings that she regularly uses in the living room, perhaps they could be moved into the bedroom too (excluding, of course, any electronic media devices).

Tuck your daughter into bed when she's drowsy and relaxed, say your good-nights, and leave the room. If she gets out of bed, try the "odd jobs" technique (see Chapter 5, "'Odd Jobs' to Foster Independent Sleeping," on page 76). If she wants to be in the living room to stay up with the adults, explain that it's bedtime and her bedroom is for bedtime, while the living room is for daytime. In time, your daughter will form positive sleep associations (see Chapter 1, "The Importance of Sleep Associations," on page 13) in her bedroom and learn to fall asleep there in preference to taking over the living room for sleep.

Night Terrors

Night terrors are among the most common causes of sleep disturbance (see Chapter 11). They tend to begin at age 4 or 5 years. Night terrors are a category of parasomnias; they mostly occur during non-dreaming (ie, non-REM) sleep, and the child generally has no memory of them. They usually start within 2 hours of going to sleep and last for 5 to 15 minutes. Because night terrors generally occur during deep sleep, and because deep sleep is increased when the child is overtired, night terrors occur most often when a child's sleep schedule has been disrupted or when she is overtired. Night terrors are not associated with emotional problems while awake.

In a night terror, your preschooler will be in bed, will seem to be upset, and may kick and scream out (for example, "No, no!" or "I can't!"). At the same time her eyes will be wide open, but she won't respond to you. You may try to console her without success. This night terror can be very disturbing to parents—much more disturbing than you or your spouse may be used to. Your child certainly may not be behaving like the child you know.

Accept that these nighttime episodes are part of normal development. Calm reassurance and comfort are usually all that she needs. In the meantime, when night terrors occur, hold your child not only to comfort her ("You're fine; Mommy and Daddy are here") but to keep her from hurting herself. Do not try to shake her awake to ask what's wrong; this will only agitate or confuse her. Typically, after 10 to 30 minutes, your child will settle down and go back to sleep. The following morning, she probably won't remember anything about what happened the night before. Most children grow out of these conditions after the early years of childhood.

Some children may have only one episode of night terrors in their lives, while others have several recurrences. If night terrors take place frequently, this may be a sign that your child is not getting enough sleep or is getting overtired during the day. In most cases, the best strategy is to just wait them out. Always remain calm. They'll tend to disappear on their own as children become older.

TOOTH GRINDING

Many children grind their teeth with a loud, grating sound while asleep. Tooth grinding (or bruxism) is very common, particularly in toddlers and preschoolers. In most children, it goes away by 6 years, but some continue to grind their teeth into adolescence and even adulthood. Tooth grinding doesn't mean that your child is having a nightmare or reliving a frustrating event from the daytime. Some causes of tooth grinding include pain (for instance, from an ear infection or teething) and improper alignment of the teeth. Although stress and anxiety can also increase tooth grinding, there is no connection between tooth grinding and problems of behavior or personality. Since it usually goes away before the permanent teeth are in, in most cases it is unlikely to damage the teeth; however, if you have any concerns, check with your child's dentist and mention it at each regular dental checkup.

Dietary Changes

Changes in diet can cause sleep changes too. If your child is having frequent arousals, try giving the main meal earlier and avoid foods with a high caloric content in the evening hours immediately before bed. However, a drink of water or warm milk before brushing her teeth may be a soothing part of her bedtime routine. You should also limit the amount of caffeinated beverages that your preschooler drinks, which can keep her awake well past bedtime. (For more about foods and sleep, see page 195).

A 3-YEAR-OLD WAKING TO NURSE

My son just turned 3 years old and still is not sleeping through the night because he wakes up to breastfeed. How do I stop this?

The decision to stop breastfeeding is a highly personal one and varies considerably according to cultural customs and individual preferences. You can be reassured that by age 3 your child should be getting all the nutrients and calories he needs from a varied and balanced diet. He is waking up out of habit or desire for comfort and not because he needs the nutrition offered through breastfeeding. If he is falling asleep while breastfeeding, this may be a sleep association for him.

You may explain that you'll no longer be offering him the breast at night, or you may shorten the time for nursing by about 2 minutes for several nights in a row until you have reached a duration of about 2 minutes, then stop offering the breast altogether.

In either case, your preschooler will probably continue to wake up at night because this is his habit. If he cannot settle back to sleep without nursing, as he is used to, let him have a small drink of water in a cup and provide some cuddle time. Do not offer a bottle or suggest milk or juice. Your child does not need these fluids for nutrition at night, and the sugars will coat his teeth as he sleeps and promote significant and damaging tooth decay. Help your child settle back in his own bed, and leave the room while he is drowsy but still awake. He may not even be thirsty but just needs comfort that he was getting through breastfeeding. Over time you can limit the amount of time spent cuddling and simply reassure him you are there for him in case he needs you. You and your preschooler may need a little time to adjust to the new system. If you experience persistent difficulties, talk to your child's pediatrician or your own physician.

The Media and Your Preschooler's Sleep

In a recent study published in *Pediatrics,* 585 families with children aged 3 to 5 years were divided into 2 groups. One group was made up of families who were visited at their homes and were guided to replace violent and age-inappropriate daytime media content with educational and other similar programming; parents were encouraged to watch television and videos with their children. The second group received only nutrition-related mailings.

Researchers then evaluated the sleep behaviors of the preschoolers, surveying children and their parents. Their conclusion: The group who made adjustments in television viewing—particularly reducing the amount of violent content they were exposed to—had a significantly lower chance of having sleep problems.

One other important point: Televisions have no purpose in toddlers' or children's bedrooms. If your child has a favorite television program, he can watch it in a central area of your home. That way you can identify and filter what and how much he is watching and the television won't be in his bedroom to disrupt his sleep.

THAT'S ENTERTAINMENT

Our preschooler is having terrible sleeping problems. He goes to bed around 9:00 pm, wakes up at 1:00 am, and is wide awake until 4:00 am. Then he sleeps until 8:00 am and stays up until his afternoon nap. Thank goodness for the television in his bedroom!

It sounds like it's become your child's habit to watch television from 1:00 to 4:00 am after a sleep arousal, so if there's a television in his room, move it out. Keep the bedroom dark with only a night-light to orient your child. When he wakes up, comfort him but don't turn on the light, and speak no more than you have to. Tell him it's time to sleep and all his favorite characters are asleep too. If he still needs some comfort as he falls asleep, give him a cuddly toy—perhaps one of his favorite characters—or another transitional object. It may take some time for him to learn this new, more appropriate sleep habit, but if you are consistent, he will sleep through the night before long.

The American Academy of Pediatrics (AAP) recommends that children have less than 2 hours of screen time (television, videos, Internet, video games) per 24-hour period, and that screen time should be high-quality content. However, the AAP recommends keeping children younger than 2 years as screen-free as possible.

For children who do watch television and videos, there should be no viewing in the hour or so before bed. Watching television around bedtime is too stimulating. It makes it more difficult to fall asleep quickly and will cause poor sleep association habits and irregular sleep schedules. These can adversely affect children's daytime mood, behavior, and learning.

CHAPTER 8

The School-aged Years: Ages 5 to 12

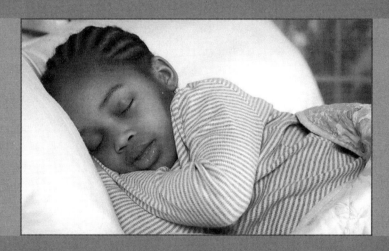

*A*t every age, children's sleep patterns are influenced by developmental, biological, and emotional factors. For example, during the preschool and early school years, children have recurrent, longer episodes of non-rapid eye movement (REM) sleep with partial arousals—which occur during the transitions from non-REM to REM phases—throughout the night. Conditions known as parasomnias—sleepwalking, sleep talking, and night terrors (also see Chapter 11)—take place during partial arousals and therefore are also common in this age group. Some children have more frequent episodes of partial arousal than others.

School Years

After a day of constant activities at school, the average 5-year-old is tired. Even if she resists the idea of going to sleep at night, it's a good idea to get her ready by giving her a bath and changing her into sleepwear for a quiet time playing a board game, reading a story, or just talking over the events of the day so that when the eyelids droop, it's only a step into bed. For a child who resists bedtime, consider placing a clock in her room. This way when the clock hits 8:00 pm or whatever time you've negotiated, she can see for herself that it is bedtime.

The amount of sleep a school-aged child needs decreases a little each year. It also varies from child to child depending on the level of physical activity and her individual temperament. The parents' activities also influence children's sleep. For example, parents who work on different shifts may have difficulty coordinating their schedules, with the result that the child's sleep is interrupted. Parents may not agree on the child's schedule—one wants to get the child to bed early, the other wants to spend some playtime with the child each night when returning late from work. But remember, sleep time should be child focused and based primarily on your child's circadian rhythm and school schedule.

Sometimes, a teacher is the first to notice that a child needs more sleep than she is actually getting. Children who regularly droop over their desks are often those who plead to stay up for "just one more" television program or for the return home of a parent who regularly works late. Children need their sleep on school nights; perhaps adjustments can be made on weekends to allow for more companionable time together with the parent whom they usually see less during weekdays.

The Importance of Good Sleep Habits

To make your child's sleep time as restful as possible, pediatricians and other physicians have developed principles to improve the sleep experience. If your child does not sleep soundly, the following sleep tips may help change that:

- Make sure your child has a good sleep environment that is quiet, dark, and comfortable.
- Your child's bed should be used only for sleep, not as a play area when he's awake. This will help him associate the bed with sleep time.
- Create a soothing bedtime routine that involves friendly interaction between parent and child. Leave the bedroom before your child falls asleep.
- Keep bedtime schedules consistent, including times for lights out and morning wake-ups, which will help your child maintain regular circadian rhythms. (For children who can read and like to do so at bedtime, be sure to set a time limit.)
- To reduce bedtime resistance, have your child go to bed when he's only moderately tired.
- Do not change your child's bedtime routine to minimize chances of demands or tantrums.
- Do not allow a television or computer in your child's bedroom. For an older child in particular (aged 8 to 12 years), enforce an electronic curfew to help him prepare for sleep without temptations. Video games should be stopped an hour or two before bedtime.
- Keep the evening household environment as calm as possible. Try to avoid family arguments close to bedtime. Avoid television programs and movies that may be violent and frightening. The same is true of active play, which can overexcite your child shortly before sleep time.

THE VALUE OF SLEEP

How crucial is it for your school-aged child to get all the sleep she needs? It may mean the difference between success and failure in school. If she gets even a modest amount of additional sleep a night—to a level that fully meets her sleep needs—she may be less restless in school and any behavior problems may improve.

Ready for Bed

Even with occasional changes in sleep schedules on weekends, many parents with school-aged children find that the most challenging time of their day is their child's bedtime. A questionnaire completed by nearly 1,000 parents of grade-school children confirmed that bedtime resistance was the most common sleep-related problem. The study, which surveyed how widespread sleep problems are, found that snoring, tiredness during the day, and taking excessive time to fall asleep were very common. Perhaps the most interesting finding was that children who had sleep problems already had these problems before age 2. (For more information on snoring and other breathing-related disorders, see Chapter 12.)

By age 11 or 12, children need 10 hours of sleep a day. During the school week, they may have to be nudged to bed to make sure they get enough rest to keep up a busy schedule of schoolwork, sports, and extracurricular activities. However, as already mentioned, a child may be allowed a bit more leeway with weekend bedtimes, depending on the activities planned for the next day.

Excessive daytime sleepiness, with yawning and napping at inappropriate times, is a sure sign that your school-aged child is not getting enough sleep at night. But behavioral issues such as irritability, difficulty in concentrating, and forgetfulness may also signal that your children has sleep problems. Some sleep-deprived children are mistakenly classified as hyperactive. In fact, their nonstop activity is a way of fighting off the daytime drowsiness that threatens to overwhelm them. Nightmares and night terrors are also more frequent among children with sleep troubles. (For hints in dealing with these and other sleep disturbances, see Chapter 11.)

Because sleep is so important, eliminate any distractions that can cause sleep disruptions. Some parents may not even be aware of some environmental factors that can make sleep more difficult. A 2010 study at Cincinnati Children's Hospital Medical Center evaluated 219 children aged 6 to 12 years who had recently treated asthma. All the children were exposed to secondhand smoke from at least 5 cigarettes at home per day. The researchers found that the greater the exposure to secondhand smoke, the longer it took children to fall asleep; these children also experienced sleep-disordered breathing and greater daytime sleepiness. The study advised that by reducing secondhand smoke, one can significantly improve the child's sleep and thus his physical and emotional health.

IS MY CHILD GETTING ENOUGH SLEEP?

If you answer "yes" to any of the following questions, it may be time to bring the problem of poor sleep to your pediatrician's attention:

- Is my child difficult to wake most mornings?
- Is my child lacking in energy?
- Does my child refuse meals because she's too tired?
- Does my child have difficulty settling to sleep because she is overstimulated?
- Is my child often irritable or cranky at about the same time of the day?
- Have teachers reported that my child has trouble staying alert or paying attention in school?
- Are our family's nights disturbed because of our child's nighttime waking?

Unfortunately, the consequences of sleep-deprived nights in childhood can linger for years. For example,

- In a United Kingdom study published in 2009, parents reported on their children's sleep problems at ages 5, 7, and 9 years. Then researchers conducted psychological evaluations on the same children when they were teenagers (13 years old). They concluded that children who had sleep difficulties (such as trouble falling asleep) as young children functioned more poorly on psychological tests in adolescence. These teenagers had more difficulty completing an effortless processing task. The researchers concluded that addressing persistent sleep problems in young children leads to improved grades and improved mental functioning as these children reach adolescence.

- In another study, this one at the University of Michigan, children who did not get enough sleep showed an increased likelihood of being overweight, regardless of their gender, race, socioeconomic status, or quality of their home environment. In this study, data were collected on 785 children in grades 3 and 6. Among children in the sixth grade, shorter sleep duration was independently associated with a greater chance of being overweight. Shorter sleep duration in the third grade was also associated with a greater likelihood of being overweight in the sixth grade. The researchers concluded that one preventive approach to excess weight may be to ensure adequate sleep in childhood.

So adequate sleep is just as important as good nutrition and exercise in making sure that your child is healthy and well.

Now, what about naps during the school years? At age 5, some children still need a daytime nap to recharge their batteries, but most have learned to pace their activities throughout the day and sleep longer at night. As at every stage of childhood, it's best to keep to a routine without being rigid. In other words, if your child is tired or irritable during the day or wants to nap, let her do so. By the time they enter kindergarten, most children need 10 to 12 hours of sleep. If your child is getting to sleep late because her preschool or kindergarten insists on a daytime nap, ask if she may simply have a rest period without napping—perhaps quietly looking at a book, instead.

Too Excited to Sleep

Nighttime fears, separation anxiety, and school worries are common causes of wakefulness in school-aged children. However, excitement and happy anticipation—such as the night before Christmas or for a birthday or vacation—are also powerful inhibitors of sleep and can lead to broken nights and daytime crankiness. Prepare for those events in a low-key way well in advance, letting the news of the occasion gradually sink in—or save the announcement until the last possible minute to minimize the buildup period. The former method is appropriate

---

WHAT ABOUT SLEEPING PILLS?

Pediatricians know that medications do not solve children's sleep problems; even for adults, sleeping pills are at best a temporary fix. Sedative medications change the quality of sleep, making it less restful, and produce a hangover effect the next day. What's more, if sleep disturbances are the result of habit, sleep medication won't break the cycle. The poor sleeper goes back to his old ways as soon as the medication is stopped; retraining is required to find ways to sleep better.

Certain medications, such as antihistamines for allergies, make children sleepy. So when prescribed, they should preferably be given at bedtime to prevent drowsiness from affecting daytime activities. Occasionally, an antihistamine may be a temporary added benefit if the child has had little sleep due to allergy symptoms. Don't give children any medications or herbal sleep preparations, such as melatonin, valerian, or chamomile, without checking with your pediatrician.

for a major, permanent life change such as the birth of a new member of the family. The latter works better for one-time events, such as a trip to the circus.

Sustained overexcitement makes children crotchety and parents short-tempered. It can rob the long-awaited treat of all its joy.

CHAPTER 9

Adolescence: Ages 13+

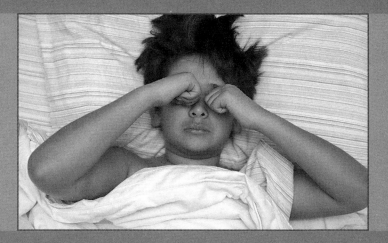

*A*mong the hallmarks of hitting puberty is a shift in circadian rhythms such that the average teen has difficulty falling asleep much before 11:00 pm. At the same time, sleep needs do not decline dramatically and adolescents typically need at least 9 hours of sleep. Unfortunately, most teenagers do not get nearly enough sleep on school days, leading to daytime sleepiness and its many consequences on health and academic performance.

Sleep needs do not drop significantly as children mature into adolescents; however, the amount of sleep that teens actually get tends to fall. The reasons? From a biological standpoint, delays in circadian rhythms (the body's "clock") associated with puberty (rather than actual age) and a drop in the sleep drive conspire to move fall-asleep times later and later. Competing priorities for sleep that help to further delay bedtime are also on the rise in adolescence, including homework demands, sports, after-school jobs, dating, socializing with friends, electronics (television, the Internet), and just hanging out. There aren't enough hours in the day for all this and sleeping too.

At the same time, earlier school start times in many communities require that teens wake up and function significantly earlier that they had to in elementary school. Squeezed between late bedtimes and early wake times, the average adolescent gets far less than the 9+ hours they need. Average sleep amounts in teens during the week are closer to 7 hours and by the time senior year rolls around, may be considerably less. The most common sleep problem in teenagers, therefore, is chronic insufficient sleep. Typically, adolescents then try to pay back the accumulated "sleep debt" by sleeping in longer on weekends. Trying to "catch up" on weekends is a problem for a number of reasons. First, it does not help performance during the school week. Second, the weekend shift in bedtimes and wake times tends to exacerbate the normal adolescent sleep/wake delay; this results in a situation similar to chronic jet lag, as the teen struggles to shift her sleep patterns back and forth. Some teens even develop a sleep disorder called delayed sleep phase (see "Insomnia" on page 131) in which the biological shift in sleep patterns becomes even more pronounced, leading to extreme difficulty falling asleep and waking up at the desired times and consequent significant daytime sleepiness and impairment.

Lack of adequate sleep can affect your teenager's ability to concentrate and impair performance academically and in sports (increased injuries). It can reduce her alertness during the waking hours. Other sleep problems, described elsewhere in this chapter, may also appear for the first time during the teen years.

Hormones and Sleep

Throughout childhood, growth hormone is secreted in regular pulses around the clock, with the highest blood levels occurring during stage 3 sleep. However, a unique characteristic of adolescence is a surge in the output of growth hormone and gonadotropins—the hormones that regulate the development and function of the sexual organs—at the end of each sleep period.

Sleep Problems and Issues in Adolescence

Excessive sleepiness among teenagers is common and is generally due to lack of sleep. This lack of sleep can have a major effect on physical health, school performance, test scores, and mood. There is research showing that there is an increase in sleep disturbances and complaints in the adolescent years, and a report issued by the American Academy of Pediatrics listed a number of causes of such sleep issues, including

- Varying and irregular sleep/wake times. As children get older, bedtime gets later on school and nonschool days. In addition, waking time on nonschool days also gets later as children get older. As noted previously, this often results in disrupting circadian rhythms and daytime symptoms similar to jet lag (confusion, irritability, physical complaints like headaches and abdominal discomfort)
- Relaxed parental control of bedtimes. As children get older, parents place more emphasis on helping children get up in the morning as opposed to helping them go to sleep. The marked difference in weekday versus weekend schedules can greatly disrupt circadian regulation of hormones associated with feelings of alertness and well-being.
- Changing school start times. Students who start school at 7:30 am or earlier obtain less total sleep on school nights than children who start school after 8:00 am.

- Part-time jobs. Students who work at least 20 hours a week go to bed later at night, sleep fewer hours per night, oversleep more often in the morning, and fall asleep more in class than those who do not work or who work fewer than 20 hours per week.

TEENAGE SLEEP BINGES
Adolescents may make up for inadequate sleep and erratic weekday sleep schedules by "bingeing" on sleep during weekends. It's not unusual for a teenager to sleep until noon and follow up with periodic naps over the course of a weekend. However, this can make it more difficult during school days for her to wake up in the mornings. It's important to try to create a more consistent sleep schedule. Make a rule that your teenager cannot sleep later than 10:00 am on the weekends. This will make the rest of the week much easier.

Other causes for daytime sleepiness include

Insomnia

Insomnia is a broad term used to describe a wide range of complaints relating to sleep. These include decreased sleep quality or quantity, trouble getting to sleep, and trouble maintaining sleep. In some cases, insomnia is a symptom of another underlying medical or psychological disorder, and in other cases there is no apparent physiologic cause. When insomnia involves early morning waking, the teenager may be suffering from depression or anxiety. The major insomnia complaint in adolescents is difficulty getting to sleep. In this age group, a major cause of this type of insomnia is delayed sleep phase disorder or DSPS. Delayed sleep phase disorder is a circadian-based disorder in which an individual's internal circadian pacemaker is not in synch with external or environmental time. An important "biomarker" of the circadian system is the secretion pattern of the hormone melatonin, which in normal cases begins in the early evening. In teens with DSPS, the onset of melatonin secretion is also delayed. Because light suppresses melatonin, environmental exposure in the evening to even fairly dim light (like from a television or computer screen) may further delay melatonin secretion and thus make it more difficult to fall asleep. Teens with DSPS typically have difficulty beginning and ending sleep at a "normal" time and prefer later sleep times (between 2:00 and 6:00 am) and wake times (between 10:00 am and 1:00 pm).

What distinguishes DSPS from other forms of insomnia is that the individual is able to fall asleep and wake readily when given the opportunity to sleep on their own preferred schedule (for example, weekends, school vacations). It can often be improved if a teen adjusts his schedule and keeps to regular times for waking up and going to bed, even on weekends. (For a suggested schedule, see "A Teenager Has to Take Control," on pages 137–138). Avoiding light exposure in the evening (and increasing it in the morning) and taking synthetic melatonin are also frequently recommended to treat DSPS. In many cases, consultation with a sleep specialist is necessary. For true DSPS, consultation with a sleep specialist is almost always a good idea, as giving melatonin and light exposure at the wrong time may make things worse.

Substances or Medications

Adolescents may also have trouble falling sleep because of the amount of caffeine they consume daily in the form of soft drinks, energy drinks, and other caffeinated beverages or foods. In addition, this stimulant is an ingredient in some over-the-counter pain relievers. These may affect the quality of sleep, especially if used later in the day (after 4:00 pm). Nicotine also has stimulant properties and sleep-disrupting effects. Teenagers with sleep problems should try cutting out caffeinated soda, energy drinks, chocolate, coffee, and nicotine (or for heavy users, gradually tapering amounts to avoid withdrawal symptoms and rebound insomnia) for at least 2 weeks to see if this helps. In addition, because many food labels do not list caffeine content, it may be helpful to look at other sources, such as the Internet, for caffeine content in sodas, drinks, and food.

Many common medications may also affect sleep and sleep patterns. Long-acting stimulants used to treat attention-deficit/hyperactivity disorder, for example, may affect sleep onset and actual sleep time in some cases, while medications for depression may have a profound effect on sleep quality. Even over-the-counter cold and allergy medications may be overstimulating or oversedating. Teens or young adults abusing alcohol or prescription or illegal drugs are also at high risk for developing poor sleep patterns.

SLEEP DIFFICULTIES MAY BE A SIGN OF OTHER HEALTH ISSUES

Our 16-year-old daughter has always had difficulty falling asleep, although once asleep, she has no trouble staying asleep. We recently found out that for the past 3 years, she has been experimenting with alcohol and drugs, and a psychiatric disorder has also been diagnosed. She is now in treatment for these problems. Can sleep difficulties be symptoms of mental or emotional problems?

A marked change in sleeping habits may be a signal that other health-related issues are present. It's important to seek your pediatrician's advice if your adolescent

- Is sleeping much longer or much less than usual
- Often wakes in the middle of the night and cannot get back to sleep
- Has phases of low moods and oversleeping alternating with periods when she is erratic, hyper-active, argumentative, and sleeping little

In most cases, difficulty falling asleep occurs when one is simply in the habit of going to sleep and waking up late. Adolescents, particularly, fall into this routine. A teenager may also lie awake wor-rying about how to resolve a temporary situation or fear. In this case, gentle questioning may lead her to say what's on her mind.

Sleep Apnea

An adolescent who complains of sleeping poorly and is unusually tired during the daytime may have obstructive sleep apnea (OSA) (see Chapter 12). This condition results in not get-ting enough oxygen during the night because of partial or complete airflow obstruction. Obstructive sleep apnea may also result in sleep disruption. The typical story is that the child is a loud nightly snorer who may or may not have apneas (brief breathing pauses dur-ing sleep, which may be followed by gasping). In contrast with younger children with OSA, adolescents often have daytime sleepiness. Other features associated with sleep apnea include breathing through the mouth, restless sleep, sweating during sleep, morning headache, and sometimes wetting the bed at night. Although enlarged tonsils and adenoid tissue are often the explanation, other risk factors include allergies, asthma, gastroesophageal reflux, and family history of OSA. Being overweight or obese is becoming an increasingly important risk factor in teens as it is in adults. There may also be anatomic reasons such as an unusually small chin or large tongue. Children with some chronic medical conditions (especially those associated with head and neck anatomic abnormalities) or genetic problems (such as Down syndrome, Prader-Willi syndrome, cerebral palsy, muscular dystrophy) also have an increased risk of OSA. While being overweight clearly increases the risk, even a wiry adolescent may have OSA, especially if some of the risk factors are also present.

Obstructive sleep apnea can contribute to poor performance at school. If you notice consistent, frequent snoring or noisy breathing and your teenager is fatigued and irritable or having more difficulty in school, arrange for a checkup with his pediatrician.

Narcolepsy

Narcolepsy is a chronic lifelong neurologic sleep disorder that frequently emerges during adolescence. Teenagers with narcolepsy become irresistibly sleepy during the daytime and may fall asleep suddenly in the midst of a conversation or during a meal ("sleep attacks"). Patients with narcolepsy can also experience certain behaviors associated with rapid eye movement (REM) sleep during normal waking hours or on falling asleep or waking up.

DROWSY DRIVERS

Irregular sleep habits combined with inexperience behind the wheel too often are lethal for teen-aged drivers and others on the roads. Sleepiness is a leading cause of motor vehicle accidents among drivers aged 16 to 29 years. Not surprisingly, the American Medical Association (AMA) has expressed alarm about the role of sleep disorders and fatigue in motor vehicle crashes. Research shows that compared with sleeping 8 or more hours per night, sleeping 6 to 7 hours is associated with a 1.8 times higher risk for involvement in a sleep-related auto accident, compared with a non–sleep-related crash. The AMA has encouraged measures to increase drivers' awareness of the dangers of driving when fatigued and has called for studies into ways of preventing such tragedies.

Sleep experts recommend that driver education courses include specific warnings about drowsy driving. It is important to highlight this and ensure safety. One prominent researcher put it this way: Drowsiness, that feeling when the eyelids are trying to close and we cannot seem to keep them open, is the last step before we fall asleep, not the first. If at this moment we let sleep come, it will arrive instantly. When driving a car, or in any hazardous situation, the first wave of drowsiness should be a dramatic warning. Get out of harm's way instantly! Drowsiness is a red alert!

These include cataplexy, in which there is a sudden loss of total body or partial muscle tone (muscles are normally paralyzed during REM sleep to prevent us from acting out our dreams), often in response to an emotional trigger (like laughter). In some patients with severe cataplexy, they may collapse to the floor. Cataplexy is the most unique feature of narcolepsy. These teens may also have recurrent, frightening visual images, called hypnagogic hallucinations, just before or after sleep, or experience sleep paralysis, the feeling of being unable to move or breathe despite being conscious, while falling asleep or on waking. Oddly, patients with narcolepsy also tend to have very disrupted nighttime sleep. If your teen has symptoms of narcolepsy, you should consult a sleep specialist.

To make a firm narcolepsy diagnosis, the doctor will look for several symptoms in addition to drowsiness and will likely order an overnight sleep study followed by a series of 20-minute nap "opportunities" on the day after the sleep study, called the Multiple Sleep Latency Test. Patients with narcolepsy will fall asleep very quickly and immediately go into REM sleep during the naps.

Although narcolepsy can be seen in very young children, it is more likely to occur in adolescence and early adulthood. Narcolepsy is a lifelong condition and requires lifelong treatment to relieve symptoms. In some cases, the sleepiness becomes less intense over time and some symptoms disappear altogether for a period, even without treatment. Treatment consists of stabilizing sleep schedules, regular naps, and medications to optimize daytime alertness.

A DIFFERENT APPROACH TO DEALING WITH NIGHTMARES

Sleep researchers have developed methods that may help older children and adolescents to diminish scary dreams. Children who had frequent nightmares were instructed by sleep researchers to close their eyes while awake, remember their nightmares, and consciously change the course of the nightmare from a frightening ending to a happy one. After only a few sessions of this, the children's nightmares began to follow the pleasant scenarios they had rehearsed during daytime sessions. This technique may be worth trying for a child who often has upsetting dreams but should only be done under the guidance of a sleep specialist or a specialist in cognitive-behavioral therapy.

Sleepwalking

Sleepwalking can be a sleep issue for teens. It is not associated with behavior or personality problems or a symptom of emotional stress. Still, many people tend to sleepwalk when they are feeling stressed, such as at school examination time. It is important to recognize that one of the most important triggers of sleepwalking is insufficient sleep. Your body compensates for not getting enough sleep by increasing the percent of time in deep sleep, and sleepwalking occurs exclusively during deep sleep. This is the reason that sleepwalking, which usually disappears by adolescence, may recur in a sleep-deprived teen.

Do not wake a sleepwalker. While a chronic sleepwalker should be watched carefully so she doesn't injure herself, it's best to gently guide your child back to bed. And when she wakes in the morning she'll have no memory of the event. For more information on sleepwalking, see Chapter 11.

Night Owls

As mentioned earlier, circadian rhythms may change during adolescence. There can be a genetic tendency for a preference for alertness in the morning versus the evening. Teenagers may become more night owls, not becoming sleepy until later in the evening and needing to sleep later in the morning. Further complicating the matter, teenagers don't like to be told what to do, and many parents, respecting their children's urge toward independence, tend to hold back advice.

TIPS FOR TEENS
A few strategies to help your teen catch extra winks include • Maintaining a regular study schedule • Powering down all electronic devices earlier in the evening, especially the hour before bed • Eliminating or cutting down on caffeine, especially 3 to 5 hours before trying to fall asleep

If an erratic sleep schedule is causing problems with school and family activities, you may ask your teenager where she thinks the problem lies. You may also suggest that she must find it difficult to fall asleep if she is watching late-night television, surfing the Internet, or engaging in social media. You can even lead her toward a solution by explaining how to shift the sleep phase back, and you can provide the tools she needs, such as a clock radio and a loud alarm. However, if the program is going to work, your teenager has to want to change and be prepared to take responsibility for following a new sleep schedule, including weekend wake-ups, on her own.

Occasionally, an adolescent may adopt a late sleep phase to cover up a deeper problem such as bullying or a learning disability. If your teenager is having problems with schoolwork or social issues along with a change in her sleep schedule, arrange an appointment with your pediatrician. An adolescent may talk more freely with an impartial health professional than with a family member. Your pediatrician will also be able to recommend an appropriate course of action.

A TEENAGER HAS TO TAKE CONTROL

Our daughter, age 13, goes to bed every night around 9:00 pm but doesn't fall asleep until 2:00 or 3:00 am. She says it doesn't bother her because she often uses the time to think out solutions to problems that come up during the school day. It bothers her father and me, though, because she is so tired during the day. She falls asleep in class and her slipping grades reflect this. We make sure she is never upset or hurried before bed, and she usually reads quietly in the living room after she's finished her homework. She doesn't want to use medication; she says she'd rather lie awake. How can we get her to sleep earlier and not have to wake her every day? We have to do this because we don't want her to miss the school bus.

Your daughter has developed a delayed sleep phase disorder (see "Insomnia" on page 131). It is possible to shift the sleep phase by keeping to a regular schedule for going to bed and waking up. The time for going to bed is not quite as important, so bedtimes may be a little more flexible on nonschool nights. The wake time is the foundation and must be consistent for a longer time. No sleeping in allowed. *(continued on next page)*

A TEENAGER HAS TO TAKE CONTROL, CONTINUED

In general, it's more difficult to shift the sleep phase in adolescents than in younger children, simply because the habit is more entrenched and the clock is misaligned between the internal timing and the societal clock on the wall. A key to success is requiring that the teenager assume control over her bedtime and waking. Most of all, she must be responsible for getting up in the morning and cannot rely on others to wake her. Put a clock radio in your daughter's bedroom and place a backup alarm on the other side of the room or even just outside her door so she has to make an effort to turn it off. Talk over the new plan with your daughter and explain her responsibilities, including setting both alarms daily. Draw up a contract and have her sign it, if this method fits your family's style. Bright light, like sunlight, in the morning within 2 hours of the wake time is also essential.

If trying this new system for a few weeks doesn't bring about at least a slight improvement, ask your child's pediatrician to evaluate the situation. Sleeping much more or much less than normal may be a symptom of an emotional condition, such as depression. Your pediatrician may raise the possibility of referral to another health professional with experience in sleep disorders.

PART 2
CHILDHOOD SLEEP CHALLENGES

Sleep troubles are not diseases in themselves but rather symptoms that can signal other physical or emotional problems. Such problems may be temporary or chronic. Almost always, treating the underlying condition brings a marked improvement in the quality and quantity of sleep.

CHAPTER 10

There's a Monster Under the Bed: Dealing With Fears

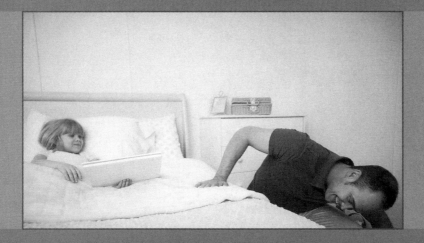

Fears and worries are normal for even the most well-adjusted child. Indeed, different stages of development are marked by certain clearly defined fears. As early as 5 months of age, for example, a baby may appear wary when confronted with an unfamiliar face. What's hard for parents to understand is that when the cause can be identified, the fear seems to be all out of proportion to what triggered it. Interestingly, similar triggers can set off fears in children the same age, no matter whether they appear to have fearful or "fearless" personalities.

"See, there's nothing to be afraid of," Matthew's mother said as she opened the closet door wide and shone a flashlight. "It's just your imagination. Now sleep tight."

The next night, 3-year-old Matthew called out, "You'd better get in here, Mommy. My imagination's back in the closet again!"

Children have many fears that they must deal with, and many of these reveal themselves in their sleep. Starting in the latter half of the first year and gradually fading away about the second birthday, separation anxiety (the fear that if you cannot see someone, he will never return) makes for frequent broken nights. During the preschool years, a vivid imagination can manifest as fear of the dark or monsters that may or may not seem to have a direct connection with the exposures and experiences of daily life. In some cases, fears can be linked directly to media exposure, including the news.

A new onset of bedtime fears may also coincide with changes in a child's life, such as starting out-of-home child care, moving to a new house, the arrival of a new baby, or a parent's move to full-time work outside the home. No matter how silly these fears may seem, they are normal and protective; they teach caution and hold children back from taking needless risks. Only in unusual cases do fears become so overwhelming that they interfere with children's development.

At some point, most children have recurrent episodes of fearfulness that disrupt sleep. Fears are often at the root of the most common sleep problems: resistance at bedtime, trouble falling asleep, and nightmares. (For more about nightmares and night terrors, see Chapter 11.) Although fears may upset children at any age, psychologists have charted 2 normal peaks in

TYPICAL FEARS AT DIFFERENT DEVELOPMENTAL STAGES	
Infancy	Loud noises, falling, separation from parents, strange faces, sensory overload
Preschool	Animals, the dark, separation, imaginary monsters, going to school (change; fear of the unknown)
School years and adolescence	Family fights, discipline, social rejection, not performing well (school, sports), war, school violence, crime, family concerns, issues related to sexual development

the frequency and intensity of fears during childhood: the first at around 5 to 6 years, and another around 9 to 11 years.

Sleep disruption due to fear is generally a normal, temporary stage in children's development. When children have learned to deal with fear, they return to their previous patterns of sleeping—good or bad. Your goal as a parent is to bolster your child's confidence so that he can sleep in his own bed without fear of harm. The way you achieve this is different from the approach you use to establish good sleeping habits or correct poor ones. A child who is frightened needs more time and attention than one who is merely testing the limits of his parents' patience. It's important to judge where to draw the line in dealing with fears to promote good sleeping habits. If your child's sleep pattern was unsatisfactory before the start of the fear phase, you will have to continue working to improve it after he has mastered the fear.

How Fears Are Manifested

Nighttime fears emerge in various ways. They are often the reason for bedtime resistance; children may dawdle, find distractions, or simply refuse to go to bed. Many children manage to put off the worst of their fears until their parents leave the bedroom or the lights are turned off. One child may come right out and say she's afraid of monsters behind the curtains, while another comes up with delaying tactics when it's time for bed. Some children

---

FAIRY TALES—PERHAPS NOT FOR THE AVERAGE YOUNG CHILD

Fairy tales, most of which originated in ancient times as entertainment for adults to pass the evenings, are notorious for triggering frightening images in young imaginations at bedtime. The moral lessons they convey, while valid and timeless, are often couched in earthy parables that are hard for young minds to break down and absorb. For children of any age who are prone to fears and nightmares, choose reading material carefully and avoid challenging tales that may conjure up scary images after dark.

---

frequently misbehave or throw tantrums as bedtime approaches. Others appear extremely restless once they get into bed; this may be a reaction to intrusive, troubling thoughts.

Avoid Triggering Nighttime Fears

- Make it a rule to turn off the television, video games, and computer in the house an hour or so before bedtime. Don't allow your child to watch violent programs or play violent video or computer games at any time; monitor cartoons and news programs to shield your child from gratuitous violence and overexciting stimulation.
- Avoid roughhousing and vigorous play at bedtime.
- Read calming stories with happy endings and sing cheerful songs; avoid cliffhangers and tales that end sadly.
- Avoid talking about scary topics at bedtime; hold such discussions in the light of day. Remember that what frightens your child is important to her, even if you think it's silly. Daytime is also a good time to talk about how you will respond to your child's requests at night.
- For a child who is unusually sensitive to sounds after dark, try playing a recording of soothing sounds at a very low volume while she goes to sleep.
- If your child is afraid of the dark, leave a very dim lamp or night-light switched on.
- If the sight of a picture, drape, toy, or piece of furniture always bothers your child at night, consider moving it out of the bedroom.

WATCH HOW YOU SAY IT...

A 2-year-old developed a fear of burning up at night when his parents told him they were putting a cool-mist humidifier in his bedroom. After he was able to inspect the device and its workings were explained to him, he accepted that it was not a "fire" but a "different kind of -fier" and his fears went away.

In addition, prayers are part of the going-to-bed routine for many families. However, some of the images of certain prayers may be troubling to imaginative young children, for whom notions of sleep and death tend to overlap. Consider teaching simple prayers with words that comfort and that your child can easily understand.

When Anxiety Is Not Normal

It is normal for children to feel some anxiety. Learning to cope with anxiety and not be overwhelmed by it is a healthy part of growing up. However, when anxiety begins to take over, your child needs help. Consult your child's pediatrician if your child seems anxious and has symptoms suggesting panic attacks, specifically

- Shortness of breath
- Faintness
- Racing or thumping heart
- Nausea
- Choking sensation
- Chest pain

Panic Disorder

A child may develop extreme nighttime fears with attacks of hysterical panic that disrupt family life. Such fears usually reflect an underlying emotional difficulty, deeper and more complicated than normal fears. In this case, your child's pediatrician should be made aware, and if he or she thinks it advisable, the pediatrician will provide a referral to another specialist with experience in treating childhood emotional difficulties. If the child's fears are centered on his bedroom, a form of desensitization treatment may be necessary. Parents and child together should spend increasing amounts of time in the room during the day, playing

---

A NEW BABY SISTER CAN BE A DIFFICULT TRANSITION

Joshua, almost 4 years old, was a smart, good-natured boy who had no problems with sleeping or behavior and loved going to preschool. He welcomed the idea of having a little sister, was aware of the basic facts of pregnancy and birth, and helped his parents get a room ready for the baby's arrival.

After the first few days of adjustment, Joshua became tearful and whiny, demanded to sleep in the crib he'd abandoned 2 years before, wet his bed, and woke in the middle of the night complaining of monsters in his bedroom. For the first time, he even resisted going to school.

Trusting their pediatrician's assurance that this return to babyhood was a passing phase, Joshua's parents bolstered his identity as the big boy of the family by making special time for him alone and reading stories that let him understand he wasn't the first child to feel shunted aside by a baby. They protected his mattress with a plastic sheet in case of nighttime accidents and let him choose a new night-light. Joshua's father stayed seated by his bed for a few minutes after the last bedtime story while Joshua drifted into a sleepy state. And to make sure that the monsters didn't sneak in after Daddy left, the family dog was allowed to sleep in Joshua's bedroom. In less than a month, the monsters and other troubles had vanished, and Joshua celebrated his fourth birthday with a new maturity.

---

games, doing puzzles, rearranging the furniture, and finding other ways to feel at ease in the surroundings—perhaps even acting out part of the nighttime routine. Eventually, with counseling, the child will agree to sleep in his own room, possibly on his own initiative. The treatment process cannot be hurried. It demands plenty of patience, and parents must take an active part in it.

What Monsters May Stand For

While monsters aren't real, the fears they stand for are real and troubling to children, even if the children themselves don't know what the monsters symbolize. For example, a child who is anxious about staying dry at night may confront his fears of bed-wetting in the form of a scary beast that comes out after dark. One who is worried about harnessing feelings of anger and jealousy may find himself under nightly "attack" by hostile creatures. Fantasies of aggression, which are a normal stage of development, may be particularly distressing after a child sees similar impulses acted out on television or in a movie.

For parents, who may feel perplexed about dealing with a fearful child, the best approach is to acknowledge fears and explain that the monsters aren't real. What helps children overcome their fears is reassurance that their parents—or whoever the trusted caregiver may be—are there to protect and comfort them.

Children may not understand the urges underlying their fears, but they are aware of the disturbing feelings such urges produce. To explain away those feelings, their imagination comes up with the all-purpose scapegoat: monsters or their close relatives. Fears usually lie dormant during the daytime, when children are on the go, too busy to dwell on problems. However, as children become sleepy and their ability to control their emotions ebbs away, fantasies flourish. At bedtime, children have to let go of the very limited control they exercise over their environment. Thus, nighttime emotions may overwhelm daytime logic, and children are less able to avoid troublesome thoughts. It may be helpful to talk about the monsters and fears during the day. However, remember that children tend to feel and act younger than their years (psychologists call this *regression)* when they're scared. Consequently, they may need a different kind of reassurance at nighttime than during the day. At times, you may feel you're dealing with another child at night, one who acts a year or two younger than his independent daylight self.

OTHERS HAVE FEARS TOO

Many children are comforted by knowing that others have fears and anxieties just like theirs. Fears, nightmares, dreams, and sleep are sensitively handled in stories such as *In the Night Kitchen* and *Where the Wild Things Are* by Maurice Sendak, *There's a Nightmare in My Closet* by Mercer Mayer, and *Ben's Dream* by Chris Van Allsburg, as well as many others. Take care, however, that the stories themselves are not frightening to your child. It may be helpful to first read a story such as this during the daytime, when your child is less anxious.

NIGHT FEARS AND NERVOUS HABITS
My 7-year-old son wakes up several times every night frightened by noises. If I also have heard something, I try to explain it to him, but increasingly, there are noises that only he can hear. He gets obsessed with the noises, usually imagining that there's an intruder in the house. I am concerned with what causes his behavior and how to help him conquer his fears. He doesn't like to be separated from me and has other fears that adults consider irrational. Recently, he has developed a twitch in his neck that he can't seem to control.
Because your child is experiencing increasing fears during the day and night, contact your pediatrician, who will evaluate the situation and may recommend an examination by another specialist. If your child is unusually fearful, becoming increasingly fearful, having more daytime fears in addition to nighttime, or compulsively repeats actions, words, or rituals to ward off fears, talk to your pediatrician.

Managing monsters takes a 2-pronged approach involving a confident, open attitude to problems during the daytime and calm reassurance at night. Children model their coping style on their parents' behavior. If you appear calm and confident, your child will try to copy you.

Managing Monsters

The best way to deal with the monsters and demons that come out at night is to reassure your child that she is safe in her own home and that her parents are looking after her. Variations on this approach depend on the individual child's personality. For some children, challenging the monsters on their own turf—shining a light in the closet or sweeping under the bed—is only an acknowledgment that the monsters are real and thus to be feared. Some children may also seize the opportunity to stretch out bedtime with challenging questions such as, "How do you know the monsters didn't hide when they heard you coming?" Other children feel comforted by such monster-eradication methods.

It's not necessary to get to the bottom of fears by questioning your child at bedtime; it may be better to save discussions for the bright light of day. If your child is upset, sit in a chair beside her bed, rub her back if it calms her, and reply to her questions without speaking any more

---

ABUSE MAKES A CHILD FEARFUL

An unusual fear of going to bed may be a sign that a child is being subjected to physical or sexual abuse, particularly in the preschool years. Your child may be too young or too frightened to tell you the cause of his fears, or the predator may have threatened harm if the child tells. If you suspect abuse or have concerns about the influence of children or adults with whom your child has been spending time, whether at home or away, consult your pediatrician. He or she will examine your child for signs of abuse and may be able to draw out information that your child is afraid to talk about with those closer to him. If abuse has occurred, your pediatrician will suggest a course of action to lessen the impact and may recommend counseling for your child and the whole family.

---

than you have to. Let your child know that you understand how she feels, but confidently and supportively reassure her. When she is calm, sleepy, but still awake, quietly leave the room, leaving the door open so that she does not feel cut off and so you can check on her, if necessary, without disturbing her.

Occasionally, your child is unusually upset and renews her frightened behavior whenever you try to leave the room. On these nights, you may find it best to sit in a chair next to her bed or even lie on the floor, if that's more comfortable. Try not to use this approach several nights in a row or you may find yourself with a whole new set of difficulties. Your child may quickly come to depend on your presence to fall asleep, whereas your goal is to help her learn to get to sleep on her own.

There are ways to deal with this problem and at the same time avoid fostering dependence. For more information see Chapter 4, "Vanishing Chair Routine," on page 62. This method of gradual distancing may take a week or two to complete.

When a young child is frightened, you may have to relax the rule about picking her up. Try to comfort her in her crib or bed, but be prepared to give her a cuddle if that's what it takes. However, keep the lights (except for a night-light) off, stay in her room, and avoid giving in to her requests to sleep in your bed or join other family members who are still up. If you bring your child to your room or let her stay up, you're putting off the moment of reckoning. The aim in calming your child's fears is to reassure her that her own bed is the most appropriate and comfortable place for her to sleep. Letting her sleep away from her bed not only rewards your child for staying awake but may also increase the fear that her bedroom is not a safe place.

Fears in School-aged Children

In young children, normal nighttime fears arise out of the child's internal struggles to come to terms with the world. By contrast, older children may be aware of many more external factors, such as overhearing parents arguing, media reports of violence, or bullying at school. News programs, movies, and violent video games can stimulate frightening images. Children who feel frustrated because of their inability to deal with matters beyond their control may suffer depression mixed in with stress and fearfulness.

REAL FEARS

My 9-year-old never had a problem sleeping until a month ago, when there was a robbery at the house next door. He used to fall asleep by 9:00 pm; now he is frightened by every little noise and can't get to sleep until at least 10:30 pm. Calming music hasn't worked and I don't want to try medications.

Nighttime fears are common and reach their second and final major peak between ages 9 and 11 years. Most school-aged children's fears are very real to them even if groundless. In your son's case, however, his fear is understandable because—like fears of school violence—it stems from an actual event, even though it didn't involve him directly.

In addition to reassuring your child, you will need to address and master any fears of your own. One way to start is by reviewing home safety procedures with your son, including fire escape routes and how to make an emergency call. If you have an alarm system, let him read the instruction manual and practice switching the system on and off. Put him in charge of activating it at certain times. If your son is concerned about his personal safety, a martial arts course could help him develop more self-confidence.

The fear triggered by this traumatic event will probably fade away after several months. If it becomes more intense, talk to your pediatrician, who will evaluate your son and may advise counseling.

A school-aged child who is losing sleep because of nighttime fears should be evaluated by a pediatrician. The doctor may advise counseling to help the family sort out its problems.

Sleep and Death

The death of someone close to your child or a pet may release a flood of anxiety and night-time fears. Children's concerns are frequently centered on the notion of falling asleep and never waking again. Such fears are fed when adults use euphemisms that talk about sleep instead of death: "We had to put kitty to sleep," or "Granddad went to sleep and he won't wake up anymore."

Your child's sense of loss may not be deep if the person who has died was only occasionally present in your child's life. However, grieving for someone closer may involve complicated feelings of sadness, anger, and fear.

In explaining death to a child it's best to use the correct words and provide the simple, straightforward facts, keeping concepts of sleep and death in their proper places: "Grandpa's heart stopped working because he was old and very ill."

Children are sometimes also engulfed by grief they cannot express when their usual care-givers leave or are replaced. A similar approach should be used to explain the departure of a familiar child care helper: "Peggy can't help us any longer because she has gone to live too far away, so now we're lucky to have Betty to help look after you." Most important in these situations is the reassurance that "Mommy and Daddy are here to look after you."

ANXIETY AND MOURNING

I have a 10-year-old who lost his father last year. Since then he seems to be unable to sleep by himself in his own bed.

Explain to your son that you understand his anxiety but that both of you must get proper rest in your own beds. Ask your pediatrician about how to help children after bereavement. Some families find it helpful to receive counseling together rather than individually.

Setting Limits

Parents become highly attuned to their children's behavior. However, at times it can be difficult to tell whether your child is genuinely frightened or just putting on a convincing show. After several nights of receiving extra attention in response to crying, a child may decide to extend the performance in a bid to keep the attention coming. This is where parents have to be prepared to set limits. Stay in your child's room while calming him. Give his worries a fair hearing, but keep your responses brief and to the point: "You're safe in your bed. I'm looking after you." Avoid becoming involved in discussions that may feed fears and prolong wakefulness.

SEEKING COMFORT FROM THE FAMILIAR

We have a daughter, 7, and a son, 3. Both slept fine and in their own beds until we moved to a new house. Now they want to sleep in the same bedroom, even though they have their own rooms. When we insist that they sleep apart, my son crawls into bed with my husband and me after we're asleep. Should I be concerned that they refuse to sleep in their own rooms?

Children frequently feel a little shaken and insecure when moving to a new house, no matter how much they looked forward to the change. Let your children have separate beds in the same room if they want to. They're not necessarily rejecting the new bedrooms you have provided. They are simply seeking comfort from something familiar; namely, each other. Give them time to get used to their new surroundings and try not to impose more changes than they can handle at one time. In a few months, they'll probably be ready for rooms of their own.

CHAPTER 11

Nightmares, Night Terrors, and Other Partial Arousals

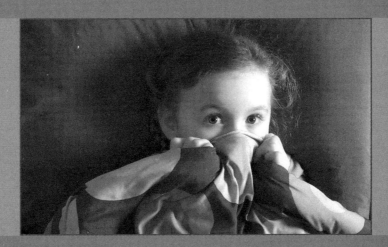

*I*n contrast with some other sleep disturbances, dreams and nightmares are normal—part of our mind's mechanism for working out emotional conflicts that arise in the waking hours.

Alex, age 2 years, whimpered as he woke up from a nap. "See elephant. Elephant have sharp teeth. It chase me. It bite my pajamas!" The toddler's face crumpled and he curled against his mother as if to hide from the angry animal.

"The elephant can't get you," his mother told him. "It wasn't a real, live elephant. You just had a scary dream. Real elephants are friendly and gentle. One day soon we'll go see one at the zoo."

Thanks to electroencephalogram measurements of brain waves, we know that rapid eye movement (REM), or dreaming, sleep takes up a good part of a baby's sleep time. In fact, during the first 3 months, babies begin each period of sleep with an active REM phase (see Chapter 1). However, we have no way of telling whether it's dreaming that prompts the little smiles, sighs, and frowns we see in sleeping babies. What we do know is that toddlers begin to report dreams and nightmares as soon as they can say enough words to do so. For many, this occurs quite early in the second year.

Nightmares are certainly upsetting. A child awakens crying and fearful, needing comfort and reassurance. Very young children may need to be told repeatedly that monsters aren't "real, live ones," so the monsters can't hurt them, and mommy and daddy will keep them safe. Almost everybody has a dream vivid and scary enough to count as a nightmare from time to time. Children and adults often have nightmares during illness, especially if there is a fever or medication is required.

Nightmares

Why Children Have Nightmares

Almost all children have nightmares, at least occasionally. They usually begin when the child is between 3 and 6 years old. Because these are dreams, they occur during REM sleep, usually in the later part of the night. The child will awake suddenly and may cry or appear at your bedside to tell you about the dream or wanting to get into your bed. He will remember the dream and if he is old enough, be able to describe it to you. It may take some time for him to fall back asleep because the scary aspects of the dream seem so real.

BEDTIME FEARS FOLLOWING NIGHTMARES

My 4½-year-old daughter sometimes has nightmares and now is afraid to go to bed. How should I handle the situation?

Nightmares are common in young children and are a normal occurrence. They are often associated with an emotionally upsetting situation. Even though your daughter, at age 4½, knows that what she sees in a dream is not real, her nightmares are very frightening. A child who has become apprehensive about having more bad dreams needs a lot of reassurance and support.

To help her relax at bedtime, you can read a calming story with her. Avoid television or computer games in the hours before sleep because the images may be overstimulating. You may want to sit in her room for a few nights while she goes to sleep. Once she is used to becoming drowsy in your presence, you can try the "odd jobs" method (see Chapter 5, "'Odd Jobs' to Foster Independent Sleeping," on page 76) to foster independence. Using this approach, find increasingly time-consuming jobs to do away from your child's room, but always return at the promised time. Leave a night-light on and the door ajar so your daughter can orient herself.

When your child's sleep is interrupted by a nightmare, give her physical comfort and soothing words. If she wants to talk about the frightening images, let her do so and reassure her that they can't hurt her. Otherwise, save discussions about scary images for daylight hours. You may occasionally need to sit down next to her while she becomes drowsy. However, avoid making a habit of it because, if prolonged, it may bring on further disruption of sleep when you leave the bedroom.

However, if nightmares are occurring frequently (weekly or several times a week), this could be a cause for concern. Discuss this with your child's pediatrician.

CHECK FOR CAUSES OTHER THAN NIGHTMARES
A child will awaken crying and fretful for reasons other than nightmares. Check for fever and symptoms suggesting an ear infection, stomach upset (gastroenteritis), or another illness that could be making your child unhappy. You may have to retrieve a favorite transitional object—a toy, pacifier, or blanket—and put it back where your child can feel it for comfort.

DREAMS ARE REAL EVEN IF MONSTERS AREN'T
A child younger than 2 years has difficulty grasping the difference between dreams and real life. Comfort and cuddle a child who wakes crying from a scary dream, just as you would after any other frightening experience. A favorite comforting object may be a good idea in these situations as well.

What a child dreams about is influenced by several factors, including his level of emotional and physical development, the emotional conflicts the child is dealing with at his particular developmental stage, and daytime events that the child finds unusually threatening. Experts stress that nightmares are normal and must be kept in perspective.

Early Nightmares

Concerns that resurface as nightmares are generally the same ones that trigger nighttime fears. Typically, worries can include the fear of getting lost, the arrival of a new baby, or a parent's temporary absence on a business trip. A slightly older child in the midst of toilet training may be torn between the desire to please her parents and an inability to resist soiling. On the one hand, she fears a lack of control; on the other, she wants to assert her independence. Dreams at this age typically reflect the anxiety such stress produces, and threatening or humiliating monsters are part of the regular cast of characters.

A child between ages 3 and 6 years has to find ways to resolve many impulses, including aggression. For example, a child feeling naturally jealous of an addition to the family may struggle with an urge to harm the new arrival. These conflicting feelings are frightening because the child worries that if her parents knew about them, they might be angry and punish her. The parents' role here is to let the child know that it's normal to have negative feelings but that there are limits to how we act on them. You need to help your child learn to control her impulses and behave in a socially acceptable manner. A toddler's gentle patting of the new baby may turn into punching, or she may come right out and say, "I hate that baby!" In this case, help her to understand that you love her and know how she feels. At the same time, show her that you love your baby as well and will not tolerate actions that could harm him.

Stories are a wonderful way to get the message across, partly because reading a story has the added bonus of giving your child one-on-one parent time that a new baby isn't old enough to share. Check your local library for books that deal with these issues in language appropriate for your child's age level. Praise your child for being a big girl and enlist her help with baby care tasks. Perhaps encourage her to care for a pet or a favorite toy as you look after the baby.

At the same time, you must help your child understand the difference between unacceptable behavior and truly wrongful acts, and she must be able to trust your example. A child who is exposed to loud arguments and violent speech or conduct in the family home will have trouble with her own behavior if she senses that her parents lack self-control. In other words, they fail to practice what they preach.

School-age Nightmares

Nightmares occur most frequently between ages 6 and 10 years, after which they seem to occur less often. For the most part, school-aged children are adept at managing new challenges as they come along. However, troubling situations at school can emerge as nightmares. Bullying, poor communication with teachers, cliquishness, and teasing provoked by lack of athletic or social skills may recur in the form of nightmares or night waking, with anxiety or depression. If your child is sleeping much less or much more than usual, complains of vague symptoms such as headaches or stomachaches, finds excuses not to go to school, or expresses feelings of worthlessness, he may need help in dealing with school problems. Consult with teachers to identify specific difficulties and arrange an appointment with your pediatrician, who will examine your child and may refer him to an experienced counselor. Occasionally, disturbing dreams may be more frequent with the onrush of anxieties and insecurities at adolescence. If your teenager tells you he's having nightmares, there may be something else he wants to talk about (also see Chapter 9). Ask about the nightmares, and discuss whatever may be bothering him.

When to Seek Help

An occasional bad dream is nothing to worry about. However, if a child frequently wakes at night with nightmares or at other times seems unduly emotional—tearful, timid, clingy, bad-tempered, impulsive, hard to control—talk to your child's pediatrician. The results of an examination may suggest the need for counseling or another treatment. If a young child is having nightmares because there is conflict between parents, counseling for the whole family may be advised.

TOILET TRAINING SHOULDN'T BE A NIGHTMARE

If frequent nightmares are disturbing your toddler during toilet training, take the pressure off. You may need to take a break from working on the toilet training. While you are toilet training, be sure that you're offering praise when your child is successful and that you are not making him feel badly if he is not. In addition, it may be helpful for your child to relax with "messy" play such as finger paints, water, and modeling clay.

LIMIT YOUR CHILD'S EXPOSURE TO SCARY IMAGES

Monitor your child's screen time, including news broadcasts, videos, movies, television programs, and video games. Although your child may seem to enjoy such shows in the daytime, the images can bring on anxiety and nightmares later on, when she has time to reflect on them. During the day, talk with your child about what she considers scary; she may decide on her own that she prefers not to watch these types of shows. If not, you can decide what is most appropriate for her to watch.

Partial Arousals (Parasomnias): Sleepwalking, Sleep Talking, Night Terrors, and Confusional Arousals

Children's sleep is punctuated by episodes of partial arousal. The spell of sleep is not fully broken by the internal arousal switches that signal the end of the first 2 sleep cycles of the night. In almost all cases, partial arousals are of no consequence. However, the form they take and their significance, if any, vary according to a child's age, health, and development. Sleep walking, sleep talking, night terrors, and confusional arousals are all episodes of partial arousal. They occur during deep sleep; because children have more deep sleep when they're overtired, these episodes are more common when the child has had a very active day or is sleep-deprived. (See chart on page 165.)

After children fall asleep, they rapidly pass into non-REM sleep, the deepest form of non-dreaming sleep (also see "Human Stages of Sleep and Sleep Cycles" in the Overview on page xxii). This phase, called the *first sleep cycle,* lasts from 60 to 90 minutes. The next cycle involves lighter sleep and possibly a brief arousal, then ends with a rapid return to non-REM sleep. Once these 2 initial cycles are over, children spend the rest of the night switching back and forth between lighter stages of non-REM sleep and REM (active dreaming) periods. These REM periods tend to become longer with more intense dreaming in the second half of the night.

Although children in non-REM sleep may appear to be battling monsters or trying to escape from tight situations, they are not having dreams they will remember. Sleep experts believe that during the transition from one sleep cycle to another, the body's deep-sleep and waking systems are both active at the same time. In this state, sleepers are said to be in a state of partial arousal. Children may talk, move, and walk at these times. They may sit up, look around, and appear frightened and upset, but they do not communicate in any meaningful way. Although a child may look as if she's awake, she is still sleeping; she cannot perform actions that involve higher brain functions, such as reading or working on a puzzle. A child will not remember what happened during this state. By contrast, during REM sleep, the body is virtually paralyzed—the dreamer cannot sit up, move, walk, or talk—but the mind is actively involved in dreaming. The dreams we remember are those that occur during this state. Perhaps the near-paralysis is a safety device—nature's way of making sure we don't injure ourselves while acting out or trying to escape from alarming images.

Partial arousals with night terrors or sleepwalking may run in the family. However, in any child, physical stress (such as sleep deprivation or fever) or emotional stress (such as a change in family routine) can trigger these partial arousals. Sleep experts affirm that night terrors, sleepwalking, and other forms of episodic partial arousal in children up to age 5 or 6 years are almost never signs that something is seriously amiss. However, when such episodes appear for the first time in an older child or occur with unusual intensity, they may be tied to underlying emotional issues and treatment may be required.

A child who is having nightmares and sleep disturbances should be helped to calm down, then led back to her own bed. Although she may protest at first, eventually she will be happier—and the whole family will sleep better—if parents set limits and stick to them.

Night Terrors

Night terrors are seen most often in preschoolers and early school-aged children. They may occur in toddlers, but they generally do not occur in babies. They often look like nightmares (the child wakes up from sleep, looking scared and crying) but are actually not that upsetting for the child. The child is not fully awake and usually does not remember the episode.

During a night terror, a child cries or screams and thrashes around the bed. Her eyes are usually wide open and her facial expression is strange. One reason that parents find such partial arousals upsetting is that their child looks and acts so differently from her usual self. Her heart is racing and she may be drenched in sweat. Her movements may be so odd and forceful that the parents call their pediatrician to report an epileptic seizure. The parents' natural urge is to pick the child up and wake her out of what seems to be a bad dream. However, a child in the midst of a night terror does not calm down when parents intervene. Even though she may have called out their names, she probably will not respond to their touch and will become even more agitated when they try to rouse her.

Night terrors are much worse for parents than for the child. Even though a child may scream in apparent fear or call out, "No, no!" or "I can't!" she may not be having a nightmare and will certainly remember nothing on waking. Episodes of night terrors last, on average, between 5 and 30 minutes, tend to occur early in the night, and may recur several times in the same night. After an episode is over, the child will probably calm down—if she has awoken—and fall back to sleep.

If you are able to wake your child from a night terror, your own nervousness may upset her and prevent her from settling back to sleep. Questioned closely, she may make up a nightmarish dream to satisfy you and end up believing it herself. Finally, when a somewhat older child awakens suddenly with a pounding heart and other sensations she associates with fear, she may falsely "remember" a dream to explain the feelings to herself. Try to stay calm and don't try to awaken your child in the grip of night terrors. Simply allow the episode to run its course.

Some children have night terrors repeatedly, whereas others have only a single episode. Even recurrent night terrors disappear naturally, without treatment, as the child matures.

DEALING WITH NIGHT TERRORS

The best way to deal with night terrors is

- Don't try to awaken your child during a night terror.
- Gently hug or stroke your child, if she will tolerate the contact.
- Don't shake your child, question her, or try to offer comfort except for a cuddle and a whispered, "I'm here."
- Keep the lights dim and speak quietly.
- Wait out the episode and stay with your child until she has calmed down and is settling for sleep.
- Remove hazardous or unstable objects to prevent injury in case your child walks during a terror; check the rest of your home for safety.
- Some children have night terrors when they are overtired. Putting your child to bed about half an hour earlier may help prevent night terrors.

COMPARING CHILD PARASOMNIAS				
	Nightmares	**Night terrors**	**Sleepwalking**	**Confusional arousals**
How many children it affects	Almost all	Less than 10%	Less than 20%	Less than 20%
Age when it is most common	Between 6 and 10 years	Between 4 and 12 years	Between 8 and 12 years	Younger than 5 years
Time when it tends to occur	Last half of night	First half of night	First half of night	First half of night
Primary emotion	Fear	Fear and confusion	Confusion	Confusion
Behavior	Wakes up suddenly	Sits up and screams	Gets out of bed and walks	Sits up and stares ahead, thrashes around in bed
Appearance	Afraid and alert	Terrified and confused, shaking and sweating	Calm	Agitated and confused
Sounds	Cries and describes a dream	Loud scream or cry	Quiet	Confused speech, cries or yells
Response	Seeks com-forting	Unre-sponsive or resists comforting	Unresponsive	Agitated and resists comfort-ing
Return to normal sleep	Delayed	Rapid	Rapid	Rapid
Memory of the event	Clear recall	No recall	Little or no recall	Little or no recall

Source: http://www.sleepeducation.com/news/2012/11/11/comparing-child-parasomnias

Sleepwalking

Sleepwalking, like night terrors and sleep talking, occurs when a child wakes incompletely out of non-dreaming sleep. About 15 out of every 100 children between ages 6 and 16 years, walk in their sleep from time to time. It can be alarming for parents to see their child wandering about, apparently awake but unresponsive. However, when sleepwalking occurs and ends before adolescence, it generally is not associated with problems of behavior or personality. Although sleepwalking is not necessarily a symptom of emotional stress, many sleepwalkers tend to make their rounds more often when they are feeling stressed, such as at school examination time.

Children usually begin their nighttime rambles within 2 to 3 hours after falling asleep. The gait may be hesitant or stumbling, and the child's walking is usually aimless, although a sleepwalker may also perform other actions such as dressing, opening doors and drawers, urinating (sometimes in a place other than the toilet), and raiding the refrigerator. An episode may last as long as half an hour.

There's no need to rouse a sleepwalker. In fact, if you try to do so, your child will be disoriented and, as with night terrors, may become distressed on waking. Better to gently guide him back to bed. He'll wake up in the morning with no memory of the event.

Confusional Arousals

Confusional arousals are what they sound like: the child appears awake and very confused. She may look at you but not recognize you. She may say things that make no sense, yell, and thrash around. Confusional arousals are similar to and often look like night terrors, but with confusional arousals, the child is just confused, not scared. These episodes usually occur in the first half of the night and last for 5 to 15 minutes, but for some children they can last longer. Like with night terrors, the child will usually not remember the event when she wakes up later. There is nothing that you need to do when a confusional arousal occurs; actually, trying to comfort or touch your child make make her more upset. Confusional arousals are quite common, with 1 in 5 children experiencing at least one of these episodes. Children start to outgrow these at around 5 years of age.

Sleep Talking

In contrast with sleepwalking, night terrors, and confusional arousals, so many children and adults talk, laugh, and cry out in their sleep that talking in one's sleep is not considered a sleep problem or even unusual behavior. As with sleepwalking, children do not talk during the active-dreaming REM sleep periods but instead while crossing over between non-REM and REM phases. Although a sleep talker may appear to respond to questions, he is not aware and should not be held accountable for anything he says. A sleep talker retains no memory of the event and it is pointless to question him the next morning, even though you may be under the impression you shared a conversation with him.

Bed-wetting

Most children are fully toilet trained between ages 3 and 4, managing to stay dry at night about 6 months to a year after achieving daytime control over urination. However, as many as 15% of children continue to wet the bed up to age 5 or even later. Bed-wetting usually occurs during non-dreaming sleep. Boys are more likely to wet the bed to an older age than girls. In most cases, the child is simply a bit later than average in developing the ability to wake up when he senses his bladder is full. The problem generally clears up as the child matures.

Persistent bed-wetting tends to run in families; 15% to 20% of children who wet the bed have a family history of bed-wetting. In fact, if both parents wet the bed as children, there's a greater than 50% chance that their child will wet the bed to an older age. Researchers suspect, therefore, that bed-wetting is linked to a genetic trait. This can influence when the child is likely to stop wetting the bed.

Not all children who wet the bed have problems of night waking. Indeed, most of them are described by their parents as being very deep sleepers; they can sleep soundly through several wetting episodes a night. They may call for attention only when they become chilled by clammy bedclothes and sleepwear. Most children are not upset by bed-wetting until they start school; however, some are bothered by it at an earlier age.

If your child continues to wet the bed, ask your pediatrician to evaluate the situation and recommend treatment, if necessary. When a child wets the bed again after being dry for 6 months or longer, or if a child is wetting himself during the day, he should be assessed by a pediatrician. The cause could be a physical problem, such as a urinary tract infection, diabetes, sleep apnea, or even constipation. Some children may also have problems with their body's production of vasopressin, which is a hormone that allows the body to make less urine during sleep.

A child who has been dry may wet the bed again when faced with a stressful situation. Typical stress triggers include starting school for the first time, a new baby in the family, or discord between parents. If your normally dry child wets the bed during a time of stress, reassure him, provide the emotional support he needs, and try to reduce the stress. If the bed-wetting persists longer than 2 weeks or you cannot identify the source of stress, arrange an appointment with your pediatrician to see if further attention is required.

If your child wets the bed, don't make a fuss about it. Protect the mattress with a moisture-proof sheet. When accidents occur, let your child help with changing the bedclothes, but

---

BED-WETTING IN A 9-YEAR-OLD

My 9-year-old son wets his bed. His father also wet until fifth grade. I know that my son needs to sleep, but I worry about him lying in a wet bed all night. I used to get him up to go to the bathroom, but it made for very unrestful nights. How do I best handle this situation?

If your school-aged son is not upset at having a wet bed, don't make it an issue; he won't suffer any ill effects from lying on a warm, damp sheet. As you point out, getting your child up to use the bathroom only disturbed everybody's sleep and probably didn't help stop him from wetting the bed.

Remind your son to urinate one final time before lights out each night. And although restricting fluids in the evening is no longer thought to prevent bed-wetting, it's probably not helpful if your child has a big drink just before bedtime. Certainly he should not have caffeine-containing drinks, such as iced teas, colas, and other soft drinks, which increase urine production.

Protect the mattress with a damp-proof sheet and disposable absorbent pads. Encourage your son to help change the bedclothes each morning just before or after his shower. Discuss with him the options of wearing disposable or washable absorbent underwear at night. Reassure him that he's not to blame for the bed-wetting; it is probably a family trait that he will outgrow. If he's anxious about staying dry at night, seek your pediatrician's advice.

don't turn it into a punishment. If he feels more secure wearing absorbent pull-ups to bed, let him do so; however, once a child has said good-bye to nighttime diapers, he's not likely to want to take this backward step. Another option is washable absorbent underwear, which may be more acceptable to the child. This also decreases the number of sheets that need to be washed. Let other family members know that teasing will not be tolerated.

Treatment for Bed-wetting

For a child who wets the bed fairly often and is not suffering from a medical condition or emotional difficulties, the following plan may be helpful. This plan works better when the child is old enough to be bothered by the bed-wetting. Before starting, discuss it with your pediatrician to make sure it's the right approach for your child.

- Talk over the problem with your child, letting him know that you understand and that it's not his fault.
- Don't forbid fluids at night, but discourage your child from drinking large amounts in the evening—and no caffeine-containing drinks such as soft drinks or iced tea.
- Remind him to go to the bathroom one last time before lights are turned out.
- Set up a chart with stars or stickers to reward him for dry nights, but avoid any suggestion of punishment for wet nights. Promise a modest reward once he has accumulated a certain number of stickers, and promptly follow through with the reward.

Most children are helped by this method of positive reinforcement. If there's no improvement after 3 months, talk to your pediatrician again to plan the next phase of treatment. A bed-wetting alarm is the most effective and long-lasting treatment. Medication to alter your child's sleep/wake cycle may be prescribed. Or your pediatrician may prescribe a medicine containing a hormone that normally helps to conserve fluid. Given to prevent bed-wetting, the hormone can trick the body into acting as if it has no fluid to spare, thus suppressing the urge to urinate.

A very small number of children don't seem to benefit from treatment for bed-wetting. However, almost all of them are free of the problem by adolescence. No more than 1 adult out of 100 has persistent bed-wetting. Until your child outgrows bed-wetting, he will need plenty of emotional support from his family. Counseling from your pediatrician or another health professional may also be helpful. Even if treatments are unsuccessful, your child should be encouraged to keep trying to stay dry at night by avoiding large drinks in the evening and using the bathroom one last time before settling down to sleep. As a general rule, he should avoid drinks containing caffeine, which can stimulate urination. Coffee and tea are obvious sources of caffeine; however, even decaffeinated coffees and teas contain some caffeine. Colas and many other soft drinks also contain caffeine. Check nutritional information labels carefully. Exercises to increase your child's bladder capacity may also be helpful; ask your pediatrician's advice.

BE WARY OF MAIL-ORDER TREATMENTS
Don't be lured by claims to cure bed-wetting as advertised on television or the Internet or in catalogs and other publications. Your pediatrician can supply reliable advice about treatments for bed-wetting.

CHAPTER 12

Sleep Apnea

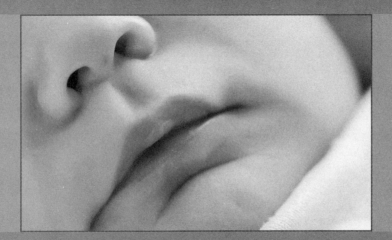

*S*leep apnea is a common problem that affects an estimated 2% of all children, including many who are undiagnosed. If not treated, sleep apnea can lead to a variety of problems, including heart, behavior, learning, and growth problems.

From a baby's first day of life, most parents are conscious of his breathing patterns. They may repeatedly check the rising and falling of their baby's chest and stomach, just to make sure that he's breathing normally.

Many babies initially have *periodic breathing of infancy,* which is a very irregular breathing pattern. Although parents are often alarmed when they notice that their baby stops breathing for a few seconds while sleeping, it is a normal condition in babies. There may be pauses in the breathing (for up to 20 seconds), followed by rapid breathing for 20 seconds. Then the baby breathes more regular breaths. There is no change in skin color. As long as the pauses in breathing are brief and your baby's color is good, it is considered normal. However, you should contact your pediatrician if you notice that your baby is always breathing fast, if the baby's skin color changes, or if the breathing pauses are long.

Sleep Apnea in Babies

While periodic breathing is a normal developmental stage, apnea—temporary pauses in breathing lasting for more than 20 seconds—is not normal. Apnea can also be associated with a decline in heart rate or a change in skin color. Most apnea in babies is *central* apnea, meaning that it is under control of the brain (in other words, the central nervous system). It is more frequent in those who were born prematurely; their brains have not yet matured enough for them to remember to breathe. Most premature newborns will outgrow apnea by the time they leave the hospital for home. Apnea is also more common in babies who are exposed to secondhand tobacco smoke, even before birth. If your baby has prolonged (more than 20 seconds) pauses in breathing or bluish skin, change in muscle tone, a fever, or other symptoms of illness, immediately call emergency medical services (911) or your child's pediatrician.

Some babies with repeated episodes of apnea may need to be treated with medication. In addition, your doctor may recommend that you use a cardiorespiratory monitor, which is a device that sounds an alarm if breathing stops for a predetermined number of seconds. However, for babies who are healthy and have the typical "stop and start" periodic breathing of infancy, such monitors are not necessary.

Obstructive Sleep Apnea in Older Children

Obstructive sleep apnea is common among older children. This condition is marked by an obstruction somewhere in the airway (between the nose and the lungs) that disrupts normal breathing during sleep and normal sleep patterns. Symptoms may include

- Frequent snoring (often with pauses, snorts, or gasps)
- Labored breathing during sleep
- Sleepiness during the day
- Difficulty paying attention
- Behavior problems

If you notice any of these symptoms, let your pediatrician know as soon as possible. Parents may be aware that their child sleeps poorly and seems tired and irritable during the day, but it may take a long time before the problems fall into a pattern that prompts a consultation with the child's pediatrician.

In many cases, noisy breathing is merely a symptom of a mild respiratory infection or allergy and will disappear as the underlying condition clears up. However, chronic apnea robs the child of sleep and may lead to daytime sleepiness or difficulty concentrating that interferes with the child's school performance and prevents her from functioning at the level of which she is capable. Rarely, severe and long-standing apnea that is untreated can also lead to high blood pressure and heart failure.

Your pediatrician may recommend an overnight sleep study called a *polysomnogram,* during which several sensors will be attached to your child to monitor breathing, oxygenation, and brain waves. An *electroencephalogram* is a test that measures brain waves. Overnight polysomnograms may be conducted at hospitals or freestanding sleep laboratories.

The results of the study will show whether your child suffers from sleep apnea. Other specialists, such as pediatric pulmonologists, otolaryngologists, neurologists, and pediatricians with specialty training in sleep disorders, may help your pediatrician make the diagnosis.

What Causes Obstructive Sleep Apnea?

The most common cause of sleep apnea is enlarged tonsils or adenoid tissue. Obesity is another common cause (see "Overweight and Apnea" on page 176). There are a number of other potential causes, such as neuromuscular abnormalities, cerebral palsy, genetic disorders (such as Down syndrome), blockage in the nose, and malformation of the face or head. Tonsils are the round, reddish masses on each side of your child's throat. They help fight infections in the body. You can only see the adenoid tissue with an x-ray, scope, or special mirror, as it is in the space between the back of the nose and throat. The tonsils and adenoid tissue grow faster than the airway does, so children often snore because they have some extra tissue in their airway and their airway muscles are more relaxed during sleep. It usually is not bad enough to cause sleep apnea and may get better as the child grows and the airway becomes larger. In fact, many children with large tonsils and adenoid tissue never develop sleep apnea. However, if your child persistently snores, particularly if she seems sleepy during the day, has difficulty concentrating, or has behavior problems, you should ask your pediatrician about it. A sleep study can tell your doctor whether your child has sleep apnea or if she is simply snoring.

How Is Obstructive Sleep Apnea Treated?

The most common way to treat obstructive sleep apnea is to remove your child's tonsils and adenoid tissue. This surgery is called a *tonsillectomy* and *adenoidectomy*. It is highly effective in treating sleep apnea but is not always successful, so it is important to have a follow-up evaluation following surgery.

Another effective treatment is nasal continuous positive airway pressure (CPAP), which requires the child to wear a mask while she sleeps. The mask delivers steady air pressure through the child's nose, allowing her to breathe comfortably. Continuous positive airway pressure is usually used in children who do not improve after or who are not candidates for tonsillectomy and adenoidectomy.

SNORING IN A 4-YEAR-OLD

My 4-year-old son snores loudly and wakes up several times every night. His tonsils look very large and I wonder if this could be causing sleep apnea.

Young children's tonsils are normally much larger in relation to their body size than adults' tonsils. However, enlarged tonsils and adenoid tissue may also mean that the child is in need of medical attention. The swollen tissues can block the airway, making it difficult to breathe. Thus, your child may wake up many times a night as he repeatedly chokes and then struggles to take a breath.

Loud snoring is not normal in a healthy child. Although there may be no connection between your son's snoring, his wakefulness, and his tonsils, call your pediatrician to schedule an examination.

Overweight and Apnea

As mentioned earlier, children who are overweight and obese are at higher risk for obstructive sleep apnea. The numbers of children and young people who are overweight or obese have increased dramatically over the last 30 years. In the United States, at least 1 child in 3 is overweight or obese.

Apnea and daytime sleepiness are only some of many health problems associated with increase in body fat. Diabetes, heart disease, high blood pressure, depression, low self-esteem, and circulatory disorders are also severe, chronic conditions linked to overweight. In addition, apnea and daytime sleepiness can lead to other problems, such as difficulties with school performance and behavior and attention problems.

If your child is overweight, he may need to use CPAP until the weight is lost. You should ask your pediatrician for guidance on a nutritional plan designed to stabilize his weight and reduce his risk for apnea. In cases of severe obesity, your pediatrician may recommend consultation with a registered dietitian with experience in helping children.

Limit your child's screen time—including video and computer games—to less than 2 hours a day. Get him moving in a program of regular, moderate exercise. This will help him to burn calories; it will also make him tired and sleep better. However, do not have him exercise right before bedtime; this may make it more difficult for him to wind down for sleep. Start with a modest goal—perhaps walking or swimming for half an hour every other day—and gradually increase the amount of time spent exercising. Try to find an activity that he enjoys because he will be more likely to keep doing it. Join him in the activity if he doesn't like to exercise alone. Even more important than fixing the current weight problem is adopting a healthy, lifelong approach to eating and exercising, which should help your child slim down and sleep better.

Remember, a good night's sleep is important to good health. If your child suffers from symptoms of sleep apnea, talk with your pediatrician. A proper diagnosis and treatment can mean restful nights and days for your child and family.

CHAPTER 13

Allergies and Asthma

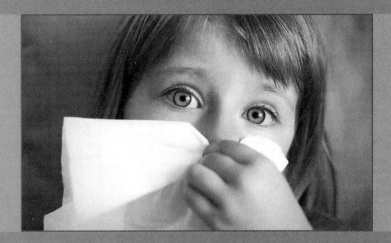

*A*llergies are among the most common chronic diseases in the United States and *typically begin in childhood. By definition, they are an exaggerated immune reaction to substances that to most people are not harmful. Genetics is the biggest risk factor for developing an allergy—in other words, allergies run in families. Allergic diseases include eczema (atopic dermatitis), hay fever (allergic rhinitis), asthma, and food allergy. Children with these conditions may experience sleep disruption.*

Eczema (Atopic Dermatitis)

Eczema or atopic dermatitis is a chronic, recurrent inflammatory skin condition with the hallmark symptom of itchiness, which can disrupt sleep. Aside from itching, skin is also usually dry and may develop crusting, flaking, blistering, cracking, oozing, or bleeding. Eczema tends to occur in infants and children who are allergy-prone *(atopic)* or have a family history of allergy.

Eczema must be treated with good skin care, which consists of moisturizing and minimizing irritation to the skin by using mild soaps and unscented products. Other aspects of skin care that must be addressed at the same time include inflammation, itch, and possible infection. Anti-inflammatory medicated creams or ointments may be prescribed by your child's pediatrician. Itch can disrupt sleep and may be treated with moisturing creams and ointments. Oatmeal baths may help soothe the itching (assuming your child is not oat-allergic; for children allergic to foods, care should be taken to use products that do not contain food ingredients). In severe cases, a sedating oral antihistamine (for example, diphenhydramine [Benadryl], hydroxyzine [Atarax]) may be needed to control itching. Infection may be prevented by minimizing scratching, which traumatizes the skin, and use of bleach baths (add ¼–½ cup of household bleach to a full-size bathtub of water). Significant skin infections may need to be treated with a topical or an oral antibiotic. As eczema improves, sleep quality should also improve.

It is important to remind families that eczema is a chronic disease and that symptoms will come and go, sometimes despite aggressive skin care. There is no cure, although for most children symptoms become less severe with age.

Studies have shown that although children with atopic dermatitis usually blame itchiness for keeping them awake, these children tend to have problems sleeping even when they are symptom-free. Many children with atopic dermatitis go on to develop asthma (see "Asthma" on page 183), and in such cases, early but as yet unrecognized asthma symptoms may be causes of the sleep troubles.

Hay Fever/Nasal Allergy

If your child's nose starts to run and his eyes become itchy, red, and swollen but there are no other symptoms of a cold or an infection, he may have hay fever *(allergic rhinitis)*. This is a reaction to inhaled allergens in the environment. The most common allergens that trigger hay fever are pollen, dust mites, molds, and animal dander.

Like other allergies, children are more likely to have hay fever if one or both parents have allergies. Hay fever tends to develop later in life because it may take several years for allergic symptoms to develop. For example, pollen or seasonal allergies are uncommon in children younger than 2 years.

Sleep problems are common in people with hay fever or allergic rhinitis because nasal stuffi-ness, cough (postnasal drip), and sneezing make it difficult to sleep. Nasal congestion may result in snoring or sleep apnea. Parents have also observed that children with chronic nasal congestion are less energetic and may perform poorly at school, activities, and sports. The degree of impairment may be related to the severity of hay fever symptoms. If you feel like your child's hay fever is interfering with his ability to sleep, contact your pediatrician.

Allergy symptoms are often treated with antihistamines taken by mouth. Drowsiness is a side effect of certain antihistamines. By giving the dose at night, you can take advantage of this side effect and help your child sleep better while relieving allergy symptoms. If your child needs treatment in the daytime, use a less sedating antihistamine that does not cause

NIGHT WAKING WITH COUGH
For about a month, our 3-year-old has woken up coughing several times a night. She doesn't cough in the daytime but begins coughing in the evening. Call your child's pediatrician, who will examine your child and evaluate her respiratory system. Coughing that is worse at night can be a symptom of asthma or postnasal drip. (Don't give her any over-the-counter medications—the American Academy of Pediatrics strongly recommends that over-the-counter cough and cold medications not be given to infants and children younger than 2 years because of the risk of life-threatening side effects. Also, several studies show that cold and cough products don't work in children younger than 6 years and can have potentially serious side effects.) If you receive an asthma diagnosis, your pediatrician will prescribe treatment and help you identify asthma triggers and find ways to avoid exposing your child to them.

drowsiness (for example, loratadine [Claritin], fexofenadine [Allegra], cetirizine [Zyrtec]) to avoid potential problems at school.

Asthma

Asthma is a chronic disease that now affects about 5 million children the United States, and the number is on the rise. Asthma is brought on by inflammation of the lining of the airways and muscle spasms in the tiny muscles around the airways. These muscle spasms make the airways narrower, which makes it difficult for the child to breathe. This can result in cough or a wheeze (a whistling sound when breathing).

In addition to wheezing, asthma can cause symptoms including

- Tightness in the chest
- A repeated short cough, particularly at night or after exercise
- Rapid breathing
- Retraction of the ribs *(belly breathing)* and collarbone

A frequent asthma symptom is a cough that gets worse at night, during or after exercise, or following contact with an irritant such as cigarette smoke or an allergen such as animal dander. Sometimes, the cough is repeated and will be followed by vomiting.

Asthma symptoms can be more severe at night, which causes children to awaken frequently and sleep poorly. Cough, wheeze, or shortness of breath that causes nighttime awakening more than once monthly on a consistent basis should be brought to your pediatrician's attention.

Several antiasthma medications, particularly those that are used when there is an acute asthma attack, are based on compounds that can keep children awake. These medications are generally not used on a daily basis. However, if your child is under treatment for asthma and is having difficulty falling asleep or staying asleep, ask your pediatrician if any of the medications might be the culprit.

Food Allergy

Food allergy affects about 8% of US children. In food allergy, the immune system tries to fight proteins in the offending food as if they were alien invaders like bacteria or viruses. Food allergy symptoms generally develop within minutes to several hours of eating the offending foods and may include hives, swelling, vomiting, diarrhea, cough, wheeze, throat tightness, and loss of consciousness. Fatalities, although infrequent, have also been attributed to food allergy.

Food allergies may occasionally cause sleep problems. Foods that are more likely to cause allergy include cow's milk and products made from cow's milk, egg white, wheat, soy, peanuts, tree nuts (such as walnuts and pecans), shellfish, and chocolate. Some people are also allergic to corn. If you suspect that your child has symptoms, including sleep problems, related to allergies or food intolerance, ask your pediatrician for an evaluation.

CHAPTER 14

Headaches, Leg Pains, and Seizures

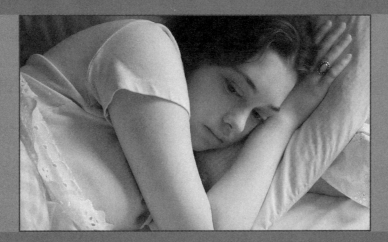

*B*ecause their bodies are growing, children need more sleep than adults. But while children need to wind down and relax as they prepare for sleep at night, a number of disorders—including those that affect the head and nervous system—can undermine a good night's rest in children.

Headaches and Migraines

Children who have frequent headaches and migraines have a high rate of sleep disturbances, including nighttime waking, daytime sleepiness, and poor sleep quality. Most adults are familiar with migraine as a condition marked by severe, throbbing, one-sided headaches and other symptoms. Children with migraines also have headaches that are throbbing and incapacitating, starting on one side of the head and sometimes enveloping the other side as well. They may feel drowsy or just find out that sleep makes the headache better.

In children, however, migraine may also take the form of episodes of abdominal pain accompanied by nausea and vomiting, or irritability, hyperactivity, confusion, and other symptoms with or without headache and vomiting. In many cases, one or both parents have a history of headaches, migraine symptoms, and sleep troubles. Researchers theorize that the mechanisms behind migraines and partial arousals may originate in the same part of the brain. Some children with migraines also have visual disturbances, called *auras,* before headaches begin.

A child with frequent headaches should be examined to make sure there is no underlying problem. Only in rare cases do headaches have a serious cause. However, the majority of children actually suffer fewer headaches and less anxiety after receiving assurances from their pediatricians that nothing is wrong. Your child's pediatrician can recommend ways to identify and avoid trigger factors for your child's headaches or migraines and will advise you and your child about using pain relievers.

HEADACHES MAY REQUIRE MEDICAL ATTENTION
If your child has frequent headaches; wakes up with a headache; has a sudden, severe headache; or has vomiting along with headache, bring it promptly to your pediatrician's attention. Most recurrent headaches are not serious; however, your pediatrician may want to rule out other possible conditions, depending on the situation.

Restless Legs Syndrome

Some children complain that they can't fall asleep or stay asleep because their legs can't relax. They may describe having an uncomfortable feeling in their legs as though there were bugs crawling inside that make them feel jumpy or nervous. It tends to go away when they kick, flex their muscles, or get up and move. Doctors call this condition restless legs syndrome (RLS). It is a neurologic condition that can begin at any age but tends to become more common as people age. It also occurs in children; one child referred to the feeling as "itchy bones." If you suspect your child has RLS, you should discuss this with your pediatrician.

The cause of RLS unknown, but there appears to be a genetic component. The condition is seen slightly more often in those with iron deficiency, a relatively common nutritional deficiency. Many patients on kidney dialysis also have RLS. Periods of inactivity, such as being on a long car drive or airplane flight or sitting in a movie theater, tend to trigger the discomfort associated with RLS.

Growing Pains

Some girls and boys complain of muscle aches around bedtime or wake up with pains in their legs and arms after sleeping for an hour or two. These aches are sometimes called *growing pains.* Although no one knows for sure what's behind them, growth is not the cause; even at the peak of an adolescent growth spurt, a child's rate of growth is too gradual to be painful.

Growing pains may consist of tenderness caused by overwork during hard exercise. Children don't feel sore while they're having fun; only later, when the muscles relax, do the pains come on.

You may not be able to prevent growing pains, but you can help your child lessen the aches. Call for periodic rest breaks during energetic play and encourage your child to take part in a variety of sports and activities. In this way, he'll give different muscle groups a workout and avoid overstraining the same muscles day after day. A warm bath before bedtime may help soothe muscles and ease aches. When growing pains are bothersome, gently massage your child's limbs; a dose of children's acetaminophen or ibuprofen may be helpful.

TIME TO GET HELP FOR MUSCLE PAINS

Call your pediatrician if your child has any of the following symptoms:

- Severe pain
- Swelling that doesn't decrease or that grows worse after 24 hours, despite first aid with rest, ice or a cool compress, compression, and elevation (RICE) treatment
- Fever
- A persistent lump in a muscle
- Limp
- Reddening or increased warmth of the skin overlying the muscle
- Dark urine, especially after exercise (If severe enough, this may require emergency care.)

Epilepsy and Seizures

About 3% to 4% of children in the United States are diagnosed with epilepsy, which is a chronic neurologic disease characterized by recurring seizures. A seizure (which is sometimes also called a *convulsion)* is a sudden temporary change in consciousness, physical movement, sensation, or behavior caused by abnormal electrical impulses in the brain.

The term *epilepsy* is used to describe seizures that occur repeatedly over time. Sometimes the cause of the recurring seizures is known *(symptomatic* epilepsy), and sometimes it is not *(idiopathic* epilepsy).

Some children experience sudden episodes that might masquerade or imitate seizures but are really not. Examples include breath holding, fainting (syncope), facial or body twitching (myoclonus), and sleep disorders (for example, night terrors, sleep walking, cataplexy).

Occasionally, *absence* seizures (previously called petit mal seizures) may be mistaken for daytime drowsiness or daydreaming. A child with absence seizures has momentary episodes with a vacant stare or a brief (1- or 2-second) lapse of attention. These occur mainly in young children and may be so subtle that they aren't noticed until they begin affecting schoolwork. Many common childhood epilepsy syndromes tend to begin after age 5, can be easily managed with medication, and usually disappear during adolescence.

Seizures occasionally affect sleeping children. Although these seizures generally occur as the child is beginning to fall asleep or awaken, they can occur at any time during sleep. They do not have lasting effects if appropriately treated.

Some medications to control seizures can make children sleepy in the daytime and thus interfere with normal nighttime sleep. Seizures themselves may disrupt sleep, yet sleep deprivation can trigger seizures, so in some cases a child may be caught in a vicious cycle in which one problem makes the other worse. Your pediatrician may be able to adjust the dosage and timing of your child's anticonvulsant medication to help your child rest at the proper times.

CHAPTER 15

Abdominal/Gastrointestinal Issues

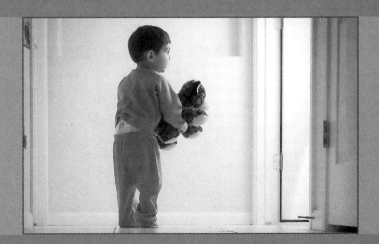

Mothers and fathers understandably become anxious when their baby or young child is experiencing stomachaches or gastrointestinal issues. These conditions can also lead to sleep problems. As much as you want your child to feel comfortable, it can often be a challenge to calm her and prepare her for sleep, leading to stress in parent and child. In this chapter, we'll briefly describe stomach/abdominal discomfort, including gastroesophageal reflux (GER).

Gastroesophageal Reflux

Children occasionally wake up with a burning sensation in their chest and an acid taste in their mouth caused by GER. A ring of muscle called the *lower esophageal sphincter* is located at the bottom of the esophagus; this muscle normally relaxes to let food pass from the esophagus into the stomach and then tightens again to keep the food there. But when the ring opens at the wrong time due to pressure or poorly timed relaxation, the stomach contents, mixed with digestive acids, come up into the esophagus and cause the discomfort commonly called heartburn. This can occasionally make it difficult to fall asleep.

In babies, GER is extremely common and usually considered a normal part of development. Most parents know this as *spitting up,* and it is rarely a concern. The baby grows out of it as her muscles mature. In general, GER in a baby is only concerning if the baby is having problems gaining weight, has breathing problems, or is having discomfort. Many babies will have a little bit of GER because they are getting too much to eat. The baby's stomach is only the size of her fist. If you feed her too much human milk or formula, the stomach can stretch out, causing that lower esophageal sphincter to open up. Extra formula or human milk that the baby cannot hold in the stomach is spit up. This is nothing to worry about. This is the baby's way of getting rid of the extra formula or human milk that she does not need.

In older children, GER may occur after a large meal or one with a high fat content. Peppermint, caffeine, and certain medications, including some used for asthma, can cause the lower esophageal sphincter to relax at the wrong time. Some doctors believe that tomato-based foods have a similar effect.

If you can identify the food that causes GER in your child, keep it out of her diet for a week or two, then reintroduce it. If symptoms recur, it's probably best to avoid that food in the future. A child with persistent GER needs medical attention. Your child's pediatrician may prescribe treatment to lessen the secretion of stomach acid or to help the lower esophageal sphincter muscle contract.

Sometimes, doctors advise that children sit upright, instead of lounging on soft furniture or on the floor, for an hour or two after dinner and before bed.

Stomachache

Children complain of stomachaches for all sorts of reasons—not uncommonly, to stall at bedtime. Or perhaps they're trying to avoid school. Or maybe their "eyes were bigger than their stomach" and they ate too much for dinner. Recurrent abdominal pain (often simply called stomachache) is common but luckily usually not serious in children. In some cases, no physical cause can be found, and the pain is termed *functional* or nonspecific pain, possibly related to emotional stress. At times, spasms in the digestive tract may cause pain. A crying child may swallow gas, which can cause abdominal discomfort. What's essential to remember is that the pain can be real, even though there is no obvious cause.

Other causes of stomachaches include the following:

- *Constipation,* although rarely a problem in younger babies, is more common in older children.
- *Urinary tract infections* are more common in 1- to 5-year-old girls than in younger children and cause discomfort in the abdomen and bladder area.
- *Strep throat* is a throat infection caused by bacteria (streptococci), with symptoms that include a sore throat, fever, and abdominal pain.
- *Appendicitis* is very uncommon in children younger than 5 years; the first sign is a complaint of constant stomachache in the center of the abdomen, which later moves down and over to the right side.
- *Milk allergy,* a reaction to the protein in milk, produces cramping abdominal pain.

FOODS FOR SLEEP

I have heard that nutrition can play a role in sleeping habits. What should I look for in the foods my children eat?

Foods affect sleep in several ways. Certain foods induce drowsiness; others tend to keep people awake; and sensitivity or allergy to foods can bring on symptoms that interfere with sleep (see Chapter 13). A young child may wake up crying if he feels hungry or may have trouble falling asleep if his stomach is overfull.

Foods that promote sleep include complex carbohydrates, such as in cereals, whole-grain breads and pasta, and legumes (dried peas and beans), and B vitamins, found in complex carbohydrates as well as nuts and seeds, poultry, meat, seafood, and dairy foods. Another sleep inducer is calcium, plentiful in many different foods, especially milk and milk products. A high calcium content is also found in broccoli, tofu, and any canned fish that is eaten bones and all (canned salmon, sardines). The amino acid L-tryptophan (an essential nutrient found in meat, poultry, milk, eggs, whole-grain breads and cereals, pasta, soy, peanuts, and a variety of other foods) also promotes sleep. It is unclear how much calcium is needed to affect sleep; it may be much more than one can reasonably be expected to consume. This is true for L-tryptophan; one would need to eat half a turkey or drink 2½ gallons of milk to get enough L-tryptophan to affect sleep.

Caffeine, on the other hand, stimulates the nervous system and promotes wakefulness. It can be found in coffee, tea, colas, and many other soft drinks. Most people are aware that regular coffee and tea can interfere with sleep, but fewer realize that the decaffeinated versions also contain some caffeine. Children are not generally heavy consumers of hot coffee and tea, but many drink iced tea, especially the sweetened, fruit-flavored iced teas sold as year-round soft drinks.

Foods with a high fat content take longer to pass out of the stomach and can cause the acidic stomach contents to flow back into the esophagus, leading to discomfort and wakefulness due to indigestion. Alcohol makes people sleepy at first but causes wakefulness later during the night; of course, alcohol has no place in children's and adolescents' diets.

- *Lactose intolerance* is when the body lacks the enzyme needed to break down lactose in milk and other milk products. Lactose intolerance is different from a milk allergy and is more common in African American and Asian children. Symptoms of lactose intolerance include diarrhea or constipation, increased gassiness, and cramping abdominal pain.

- *Emotional upset,* particularly in school-aged children, may cause recurrent abdominal pain that seems to have no other cause.

Abdominal pain that comes on suddenly or persists may require prompt attention, especially if your child has additional symptoms, such as a change in his bowel pattern, vomiting, fever (temperature of 100.4°F or higher), sore throat, or headache. Even when no physical cause can be found, the child's distress is genuine and should receive appropriate attention. Call your pediatrician promptly if your baby is younger than 1 year and shows signs of stomach pain (for example, legs pulled up toward the abdomen, unusual crying); if your child aged 4 years or younger has recurrent stomachache; or if abdominal pain awakes him or stops him from getting to sleep.

CHAPTER 16

Developmental Disabilities and Attention-Deficit/ Hyperactivity Disorder

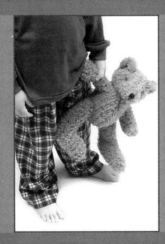

*A*lthough sleep problems in children are one of the most frequent concerns that parents discuss with pediatricians, sleep disruptions and disorders are particularly common among children with developmental difficulties. When parents better understand the reasons and management strategies, such sleep issues can often be minimized.

Intellectual Disabilities and Medical Conditions

The term *intellectual disability* (formerly known as *mental retardation*) is used when a child's intelligence and abilities to adjust to his surroundings are significantly below average and affect the way he learns and develops new skills. The more severe the disability, the more immature a child's behavior will be for his age.

For children with severe intellectual disability, sleep disturbances are a major problem and occur in more than 50% of affected children. Children with medical conditions like epilepsy (seizures that occur repeatedly over time) and physical disabilities like cerebral palsy are more likely to have sleep challenges as well. No matter what the cause of your child's sleep problem, good sleep habits are always helpful.

Other Disorders and Syndromes

Sleep problems are common in children with genetic disorders such as Prader-Willi syndrome (marked by poor muscle tone, low levels of sex hormones, and a constant feeling of hunger) and Angelman syndrome (a genetic condition marked by an unsteady gait, atypical laughter, seizures, and distinctive facial features). Children with attention-deficit/hyperactivity disorder (ADHD) and autism spectrum disorders (ASDs) also experience significant sleep challenges; these are addressed in more depth in this chapter.

Attention-Deficit/Hyperactivity Disorder

Although every child can occasionally seem inattentive and hyperactive, the term ADHD is used by pediatricians to describe a condition in which a child consistently has difficulty paying attention for periods of time or difficulty sitting still when it is necessary to do so. The child can become easily distracted, can act on impulse, and may have difficulty sleeping.

About 1 to 2 in 20 children and adolescents are affected by ADHD. Especially when children are toddlers, parents often worry that their child is hyperactive and may have ADHD. However, if you compare your child to others her age, you may notice that her behavior is typical among her peer group. Many children of that age have short attention spans and are easily distractible, and often children have significant improvements in their attention span and impulse control as they move from the toddler to preschool age range. Although ADHD can last a lifetime, it is typically first diagnosed in childhood. It often comes to parents' attention because the child is having difficulty in school.

In addition, children with ADHD can have sleep-related symptoms, such as difficulty sleeping soundly, feelings of fatigue on awakening, and nightmares. Such sleep problems may have a direct negative influence on a child's daytime ADHD symptoms and interfere with her quality of life. A number of studies have shown that about 25% to 50% of children and teenagers with ADHD have trouble falling asleep and maintaining sleep. At bedtime, these children fidget more often and become more restless and may be particularly susceptible to conflicts when they should be getting ready for bed.

A number of prescription medications have been used in children with ADHD. They may be able to help children improve concentration and control their behavior. But ironically, side effects from these drugs may include sleeplessness. Your child's pediatrician may be able to adjust the dosage schedule to enable your child to rest at the proper time.

An Australian study found that sleep problems in children with ADHD are common and are associated with poorer patient outcomes in a number of areas. In that study, moderate to severe sleep problems were associated with poor psychosocial quality of life, poor daily functioning, and poor caregiver mental health and family functioning. Compared with children with ADHD but without sleep issues, those with sleep problems were more likely to miss or be late for school, and their caregivers were more likely to be late for work.

There is debate about whether children with ADHD should use medications to help them sleep. One of the most commonly recommended sleep aids for children with ADHD is melatonin, usually recommended in a dose of 1 to 3 mg 1 to 2 hours before bedtime. While melatonin can be useful in addressing sleep disturbances in a child with ADHD, the reported positive effects as a treatment for ADHD core symptoms have been solely ancedotal so far, and there is insufficient scientific evidence to support its use. Although melatonin is an over-the-counter supplement, check with your pediatrician before giving it to your child. (Also see "Melatonin" on page 204.)

The same advice is appropriate for other supplements, including antioxidants or herbs, which may help some children sleep better. You may have run across or seen ads for substances that have been marketed as treatments for ADHD. These supplements include Pycnogenol, which

---

STRATEGIES WHEN A CHILD WITH ATTENTION-DEFICIT/HYPERACTIVITY DISORDER HAS SLEEP DIFFICULTIES

Every child with attention-deficit/hyperactivity disorder (ADHD) is different. Some children are always "on the go" during the day and then collapse at night, easily falling asleep. Others are active during the day, but as their ADHD (stimulant) medication wears off in the late afternoon or evening, they become more and more active and may have difficulty "winding down" to fall asleep.

Here are several tips that can help you and your child with sleep difficulties (some of these guidelines are also mentioned elsewhere in this book).

- Develop bedtime rituals/routines that will help your child "wind down."
- Pay attention to the sleep environment, eliminating background noises and lighting that can affect a child's ability to fall asleep.
- Make the bed a sleep-only zone.
- Establish consistent waking times.
- Chart your child's progress and praise him for successful quiet nights; consider marking successful nights on a star chart and providing rewards at the end of the week.
- In the evening, avoid toys, games, video games, and television shows that may keep your child awake.
- Any medications to help your child sleep should only be used with the guidance of your child's doctor. Some children with ADHD may actually be helped by a small dose of a stimulant medication at bedtime. Paradoxically, this dose may help a child to get organized for sleep.

is derived from pine bark; ginkgo biloba extract, which is more often used to treat memory disorders and circulatory problems; as well as valerian, lemon balm, kava, hops, and passion flower. However, keep in mind that none of these supplements have proven benefits for managing ADHD. In addition, they are not standardized or regulated by the US Food and Drug Administration and so can vary in potency and purity from one brand to another. Finally, some of these supplements can have adverse side effects by themselves and when given at the same time as other medicines. This is why it is critical that you let your pediatrician know that you're considering using these substances.

Autism Spectrum Disorder

The number of children diagnosed with ASDs has increased significantly in recent years, and now it affects about 1 in 88 children in the United States. These children have difficulty with normal communication, social skills, restricted interests, and repetitive behaviors. Their speech may be limited, and they may ignore others.

In general, the earlier that an ASD is diagnosed and treated, the more likely it is that treatment will be effective. Thus, it is important for parents to be alert for symptoms such as lack or loss of language, repetitive body movements, avoiding eye contact, and failure to respond to other people.

Studies shows that about 40% to 80% of children with an ASD experience sleep problems. If your child has been diagnosed with an ASD, manage his sleep environment and bedtime behavior in a way that does not make his behaviors worse. Before bedtime, limit or eliminate television watching and video games. Your child should also avoid caffeinated drinks. Keep his room warm but comfortable—not too hot, too cold, too loud, or too well-lit.

Children with ASDs may also be more prone to other sleep disorders, including obstructive sleep apnea (see Chapter 12), restless legs syndrome (see Chapter 14), and delayed sleep phase syndrome (see Chapter 9). Occasionally, a polysomnogram (overnight sleep study) is needed to diagnose sleep disorders, particularly if there are potentially several sleep disorders in the same child.

AUTISM SPECTRUM DISORDERS AND SLEEP

A study by researchers at the University of California, Davis, found that children with autism spectrum disorders (ASDs) awoke in the middle of the night significantly more often than typically developing children. This study involved 529 boys and girls with a mean age of 3.6 years. Fifty-three percent of children with ASDs had at least one frequent sleep problem, compared with 32% in the typical development group.

What About Medications?

A number of medications can be used to treat sleep disturbances in children with ASDs. Melatonin (see "Melatonin" on page 204) is a supplement used in some children with ASDs. Diphenhydramine (Benadryl), an antihistamine that has sedating effects, is another commonly used nonprescription medication. It appears safe and effective but has not been well studied as a sleep medication. It can cause side effects like excitation, dry mouth, and next-day drowsiness.

Your doctor may recommend one of these or another medication that can promote sleep, including mirtazapine (Remeron), trazodone (Desyrel), and hydroxyzine (Anx, Atarax).

Medications May Cause Sleeplessness

Medications can interfere with sleep. For example, those prescribed for children with ADHD are intended to improve concentration and help them control their behavior, but side effects can sometimes include sleeplessness. Some sedatives and medications given to control seizures can make children sleepy in the daytime and thus interfere with normal nighttime sleep. Your pediatrician may be able to revise the dosage schedule to enable your child to rest at the proper time.

Remember, even if you do give your child a medication to address her sleep problems, medications alone generally do not solve the problems. It's important to also use behavioral interventions as discussed in this book to help your child into a good sleep pattern.

MELATONIN

Melatonin is a hormone naturally secreted by the brain's pineal gland; in supplement form, it is sometimes used to help children fall sleep. Melatonin helps to regulate the body's sleep/wake cycle. In humans, who normally sleep at night and remain awake during the day, melatonin releases a signal to "shut down" for sleep at night. At times, doctors recommend melatonin for children with developmental disabilities. Such children can have severe sleep problems because of their inability to establish normal circadian rhythms. In fact, some studies have shown that children with autism spectrum disorders produce low melatonin levels. Melatonin treatment should only be used under the supervision of your child's doctor, who can help decide if melatonin might help your child. The doctor can explain side effects, like nightmares and nighttime waking, that occur in some people taking melatonin. Melatonin is generally considered safe but only when used for short periods. When used, it is most helpful in children who have trouble falling asleep and increasing the length of time spent sleeping (but usually not to *keep* them asleep). Of course, by sleeping better at night, these children tend to have better daytime behavior, contributing to less stress in the family.

The Road Ahead

Generally speaking, your child will settle down with the measures that are woven into your bedtime routine. Like most parents, you will develop a system by trial and error. It may incorporate bits and pieces of several methods, along with advice from your pediatrician. Above all, trust your instincts. You know what makes your child comfortable.

As you steer the road ahead, keep in mind these overarching principles.

- Understand what is "normal" and "typical" for your child's age and stage of development.
- All parents want their child to be happy. However, sometimes in an effort to make your child happy in the short term, you can end up creating problems in the long term.
- Think about what you want your life to be like in 6 months.
- Remember who the boss is. In other words, you are stronger than you think you are.

We hope that reading this book has helped you to navigate the advice you are receiving and adopt the strategies that will help you and your child get a good night's sleep and wake up refreshed and ready for work and play.

Index